Free your hair, and the rest will follow.

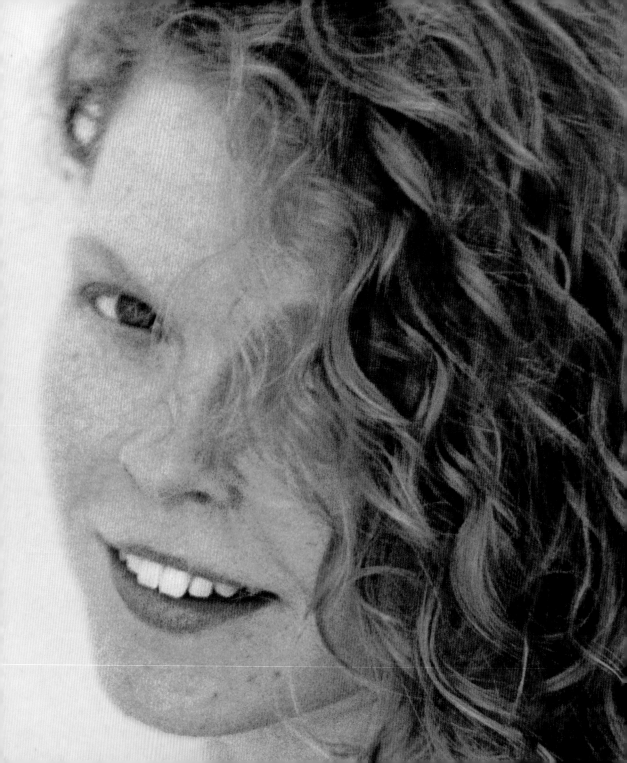

CURLY GIRL

More than just hair . . . it's an attitude

A CELEBRATION OF CURLS: HOW TO CUT THEM, CARE FOR THEM, LOVE THEM, AND SET THEM FREE

•

by LORRAINE MASSEY
with DEBORAH CHIEL

•

WORKMAN PUBLISHING
NEW YORK

Library of Congress Cataloging-in-Publication Data

Massey, Lorraine
   Curly girl : more than just hair . . . it's an attitude :
a celebration of curls : how to cut them, care for them,
love them, and set them free / by Lorraine Massey with
Deborah Chiel
      p. cm.
ISBN-13: 978-0-7611-2300-2 (alk. paper)
   1. Hair—Care and hygiene. I. Title

RL91.M28 2001
646.7'24—dc21   2001026842

Workman books are available at special discounts when
purchased in bulk for premiums and sales promotions as
well as for fund-raising or educational use. Special editions
or book excerpts can also be created to specification.
For details, contact the Special Sales Director at the
address below.

Workman Publishing Company, Inc.
225 Varick Street
New York, NY 10014-4381
www.workman.com

Printed in the United States of America

First printing January 2002
10 9

In memory of A. Dance,
and for Kaih, Shey, and Dylan

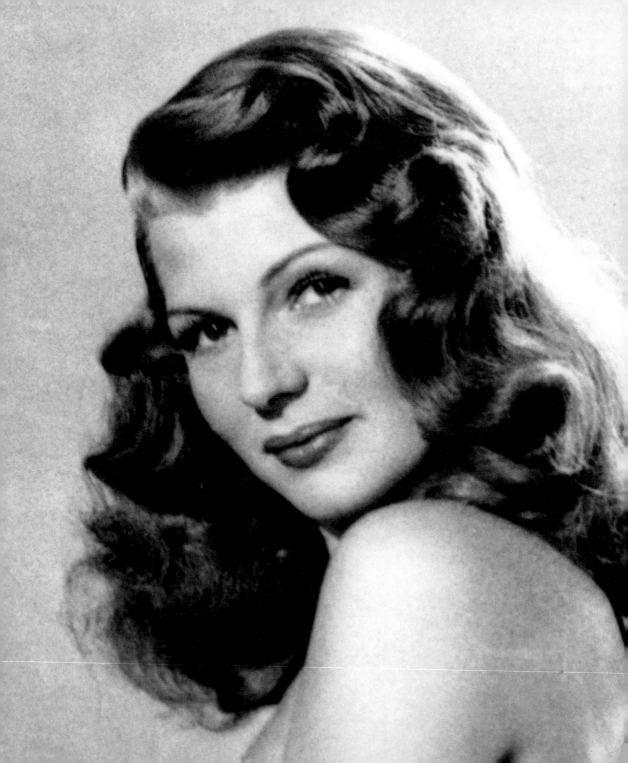

ACKNOWLEDGMENTS

Many people helped us transform *Curly Girl* from dream to reality. We are very grateful to David Schiller, Lorraine's longtime client, who loved the concept so much that he insisted we bring it to Workman. Our heartfelt thanks also to Naomi Chiel-Bolzman and Kinneret Chiel, who recognized a great book idea when they heard it and knew that we would make the perfect "curlaborative" team. Peter Workman asked all the right questions and showed such faith in the project that we knew our book had found the right home.

Our editor, Ruth Sullivan, was unstinting with her advice, her hands-on shaping to create a book that fit her vision, and in her determination to push us to our creative limits. Jessica Firger helped us sort out inconsistencies and clarify murky instructions, chased down photographs, and kept us sailing smoothly through. Thanks, also, to Paul Hanson and Elizabeth Johnsboen for their artistic vision. Thanks to Güler Uğur, Rivka Hain, Patty Bozza, Elizabeth Gaynor, and Tiffany Lee for their input and curly girl spirit, and to Anthony Loew for his wonderful photographs. Jenny Mandel encouraged and advised us throughout the process. Carolan Workman's enthusiasm helped bring this all together. She is a true curly girl. Special thanks to Carol Kramer, who gave us a schedule, a structure, her editorial expertise, and the confidence that *Curly Girl* would actually become a book.

More than we can ever express, we applaud the entire staff of Devachan for their enthusiasm, support, and their amazing ability to cope with bright lights, construction sites, and crowds of curly girls. Special thanks to Carlos Flores and Ed Fagley, who have so totally embraced the curly girl philosophy. A huge bouquet of gratitude to Devachan co-owner, Denis DaSilva, and Shari Harbinger, multitalented artists who have contributed so much love, information, color, and creativity to our lives and our book.

Henry Dreher has straight hair but thinks curly; he gave us fabulous input, shared our highs and lows, and accepted our need for creative working sessions at odd hours and in all sorts of unusual venues. We especially thank Michael and Lorraine's children for their unconditional love and patience, and for putting up with their mother's endless phone conferences and editorial meetings. Kaih, Shey, and Dylan: Mummy promises to make it up to you.

Finally, to all the curly girls, young and old, who answered our questions, submitted to our scrutiny, smiled for the camera— this book could never have happened without each and every one of you. You have the curly spirit. More power to you!

—*Lorraine Massey and Deborah Chiel*

I want to thank Lorraine, my hair spiritualist and dream co-author, for her unique vision and sense of style, and for all the wondrous twists and turns she's brought into my life.

—*D.C.*

Much love and thanks to all of my clients, who have supported me throughout the years and become my second family. Special thanks to Debbie, the best outreach curly girl.

—*L.M.*

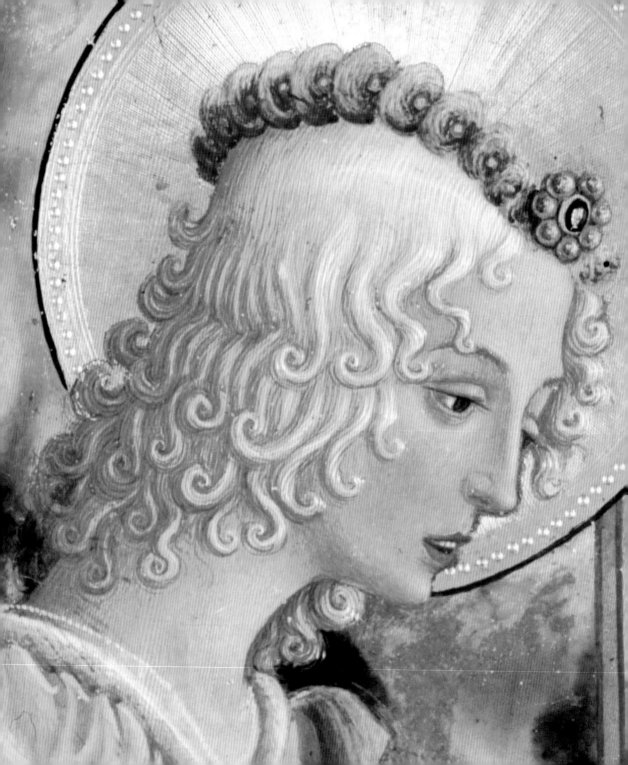

Table of Contents

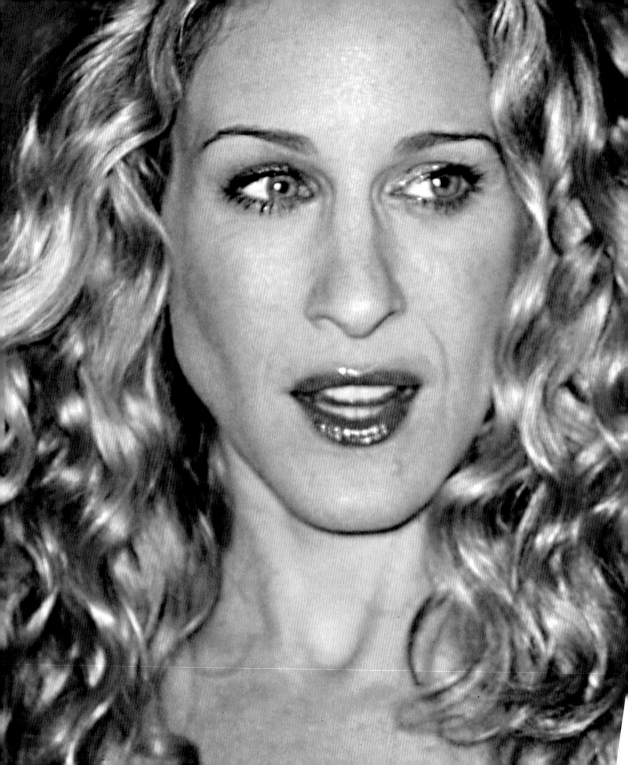

INTRODUCTION

C urls? The word sounds frivolous, too frothy to be the subject of a book. But we promise you, curls are serious business—and the horror stories you'll read in this book are shocking enough to, well, curl your hair. And so is the misinformation curly-headed women are likely to receive from hair care professionals.

For centuries, curls were considered a blessing, grace notes that added to a woman's beauty. But that attitude changed at some point in the twentieth century, and several generations of women grew up thinking their curls were not a blessing, but a colossal pain in the tress.

Most women with curly hair today have fought with it all their lives. They were teased in school and at home (usually by their straight-haired brothers). They searched for role models in fashion magazines and movies, only to see nothing but straight, lanky hair (usually blond). They've felt unsophisticated, silly, juvenile. Their hair frizzed up at inopportune moments, broke off in clumps if treated too harshly. They've imagined their curls holding them back from dates and jobs. They've been stereotyped, depending on the bias, as wenches or witches. They've spent a fortune on defrizzing products and other lotions that promised instant straight hair.

But the problem wasn't just one of attitude. There was literally no place for curly-haired women to go, because most hairdressers, especially in this country, have been just as tangled up in the hair stereotypes as the rest of the world. The catalog of curly hair crimes committed in many beauty salons is frightful:

disastrous haircuts, brutal brushing and blow-drying, chemicals that could straighten out a hardened criminal.

This book is meant to change all that—end the prejudice, celebrate the beauty of curls, but most of all, teach women with curly hair a whole new way of life. The program you're about to read is revolutionary: It will require an attitude adjustment, a straightening of the head, rather than the hair, if you will.

But the results will be astounding. Follow the routines in this book and your hair will be transformed. It will shine as never before, behave itself in public, even during typhoons, and frame your face with the world's most graceful beauty accessory, the natural curl.

Chapter One

OUR CURLS, OURSELVES

Finding Your Inner Curl

*It's your head, not your hair,
that needs straightening.
And here's how to start.*

Welcome to Curl Talk, a place where you can finally let down your hair. Chances are, if you picked up this book, you belong to the sisterhood of curly girls, women who've been fighting their curly hair for most of their lives, hiding it under hats, pulling it back, tugging at it with rubber bands, disguising it with braids, or flattening it out with anything they could find.

Depending on what era you were born into, you may have tried chemical straighteners, blow-dryers, irons, or gigantic juice-can rollers to straighten your hair. I know, just look at my picture on this page—the curls look pretty great, don't they? But they didn't always, and it took me a long time to learn to love and respect them. Now I spend most of my time, as the co-owner of a Manhattan salon, encouraging my clients to find their inner curl—an attitude that helps them accept their curls and make the most of them, straightening out their heads instead of their hair.

From the time I was born in the mid-1960s to just a few years ago, curly hair was made fun of more than it was admired. I hated my hair from the moment I was able to look in the mirror and see that, unlike my six brothers and sisters, whose hair looked appropriately lank and British, I had corkscrew curls that stuck out all over my head, making me look like Orphan Annie. By the time I was three, I was asking my mother for a straight-haired wig so I could pretend I was a Polynesian hula dancer. It was a strange request from a toddler living in a factory town in the British West Midlands. But for years I was sure that there'd been some mistake at the hospital and I'd been sent home with the wrong set of parents.

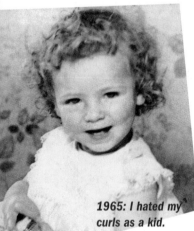

1965: I hated my curls as a kid.

I wasn't alone. As you read this book, you'll find the personal stories of many other curly girls who went through the same denial and despair I did. We all worried about humid days, when despite all our efforts our hair would frizz up. We were teased by kids in school ("Hey, Brillo, where'd you get that hair?") and made to feel that curls were inferior.

By the time I was four, I was watching the telly with my older brothers and sisters and admiring Mary ("Those Were the Days") Hopkins, a mod-generation pop star with stick-straight hair that swung back and forth as she played her guitar. If only my hair could swing, I'd think. I'd pull my sweater halfway over my head so that it hung down across my back. Voila!—I had straight hair, too.

As I got older and watched celebrities like Cher and Twiggy swing their long, perfect locks, I became more convinced that my curls were an aberration, a perverse joke played on some of us by a whimsical universe. A genetic mistake that the gods of beauty had planted in my DNA. I'd spend all day thinking up ways to make my hair stay flat and frizz-free. In my mind, the equation was simple: Straight was beautiful, curly was ugly. A sociologist might point out that for many people, this preference for straight hair was a subtle side effect of racism. Most of us have been influenced by stereotypes of beauty promoted in the last half of the twentieth century—the white Anglo-Saxon look, with straight blond hair and a pale complexion. Children could have curls—if they were golden—but they'd damn well better straighten out by the time they grew up.

I would go to bed at night, my hair tightly wound—imprisoned, actually— around gigantic rollers. I'd lie very still lest one should slip off and the curls spring cruelly and sadistically back to life.

So it was ironic, but maybe inevitable, that I decided to become a hair-dresser. I'd spent so much time fixing my own hair that I might as well try to make a living fixing others'. I served three years as an apprentice in London, then moved to Hong Kong for four years and became fascinated with my customers' straight hair. Next, I lived in Japan, where the only word of Japanese I learned in two years was *masuga.* It means "straight," of course.

Even after *Charlie's Angels* made long wavy hair fashionable in the 1970s, I kept mine short and straight. One year, I decided to wear it slicked back and short—remember that look? I think it was called a DA in this country. I was proud of it. But when I asked a not-so-diplomatic male friend what he thought, he said the back of my head looked like a "baboon's bum."

That was it. Like an addict who's bottomed out, I realized I couldn't fight my curls anymore. I started letting my hair grow. I stopped blow-drying it every morning. Meanwhile I read every scrap of information I could find about curly hair and how to take care of it. As it turns out, there is very little to be found on the subject. As the owner of a New York City beauty school told me recently, "Hair is hair, we treat curly the same as straight." No wonder so many people still straighten their hair.

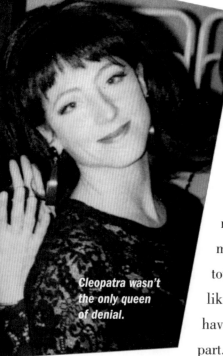

Cleopatra wasn't the only queen of denial.

But I was determined to make my curly hair work. I began conditioning it regularly, experimenting with different products, upping the amounts of moisturizers. I let it grow out so that the soft *S*'s that are my hair's natural shape had room to develop. Eventually my scalp sprouted soft curlets that grew into ringlets, then tightened into thick corkscrews that spiraled down my shoulders. This was the way I was meant to look, my hair destiny, I came to believe. And I became totally politicized about curly hair. I saw it almost like an arranged marriage—not something I would have chosen for myself, but mine "till death do us part." I vowed that no one was going to straighten my hair or my mind again. "Free your hair, and the rest will follow" became my manifesto.

Unfortunately, while I had changed, the world around me hadn't. Straight hair was still the gold standard, especially in Beverly Hills. I had moved to California and gotten a job in a fashionable salon right out of *Shampoo,* the Warren Beatty movie about a hip hairdresser. I had been working there for about a week when the salon owner returned from a vacation. He looked at me, the new girl with politically incorrect curls, and went ballistic. "Someone blow-dry that girl's hair," he shouted. I left my post at the shampoo bowl and walked. Unlike Lot's wife, I never looked back.

I moved to New York, where, for the first time in the life of my curls, I was in the majority, surrounded by people who looked like me. Ethnic-looking people: Jewish, Italian, Latino, African American. Their hair was curly, too. I no longer looked or felt like an outsider.

A few weeks ago a friend jokingly accused me of living in a "curlocentric" world. That may be true—but it's also true that we still live in a world where the WASP stereotype has a tremendous hold on our imaginations. Perhaps that explains why so many of us are still in curl denial, why cosmetology schools still teach stylists to "cut against the curl," and why so many hairdressers are intimidated by curly hair, preferring to blow it out straight rather than to work with its texture and shape. I attend many workshops and seminars around the country for hairdressers, but I haven't found one yet that features curly hair—or curly-haired models.

Pregnant, full and bouncy.

I'm trying to make up for that lack with this book and with my work as co-owner of Devachan, a salon in New York's SoHo neighborhood, where curly girls seem to find me like flocks of curly-haired homing pigeons. I've watched them learn to love their hair and work *with* it instead of against it. Finding their inner curl makes them strong, willing to stand up to stereotypical attitudes and prejudices.

Curly hair is the wave of the future. Sixty-five percent of women have curly or wavy hair. (Take the quiz on the following pages to see if maybe you are one of them.) For too long we curly girls have been at a loss

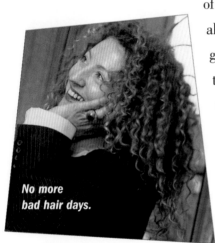

No more bad hair days.

about how to care for our hair properly or, worse, have gone through life pretending we are straight and mistreating our natural curls. I'm hoping that this book will revolutionize the way we look at curly hair. In it, you'll find a complete guide to curls, their origins, their problems, their special needs. You'll learn a radical and logical way to care for your hair, nurturing its natural curl. How to cleanse, condition, and style it, and how to have it cut well instead of sliced, carved, and butchered. You'll wear your curls proudly every day—even if you think you're having a bad hair day. I promise. It will change your life. So curl up (sorry) and start reading.

Are You a Curly Girl?

A re you still hiding the truth from the world, maybe even from yourself? Take this simple question-hair to determine whether you're a member of the curly clan.

CURLY CLUES

☐ *1. Do you often wear your hair tied back in a ponytail?*

☐ *2. Does your hair develop volume in humid, hot, or wet weather?*

☐ *3. Does your hair make you feel out of control?*

☐ *4. Do you find yourself crying after every haircut?*

☐ *5. Look at old photographs and recall how you felt about your hair—and yourself—on the day the picture was taken. Was there a strong correlation between your hair and your mood?*

☐ *6. Do you almost always have a haze of frizz around your head?*

Michella L.: *still wears hair pulled back straight in a ponytail*

☐ 7. *Do you blow-dry your hair so often that its texture is as dry and brittle as a piece of melba toast?*

☐ 8. *Does your budget for products to straighten or relax your hair exceed your annual tax-deductible contributions to charity?*

☐ 9. *Do you live in fear of humidity, sweating, spontaneous sex, a shower with your lover—or any weather or activity that might unmask you as a curly girl?*

☐ 10. *Are you almost always unhappy with your hair?*

☐ 11. *Do you worry about your hair before any big occasion, like a wedding or an important business meeting?*

If you answered yes to one or more questions, congratulations! You know who you are. You're a curly girl waiting to happen. Your hair is bristling with movement longing to break free, waves aching to curl, frizz begging for direction. Read on!

Chapter Two

HAIR
The Inside Story

*On every curly-haired
baby's head, there should be
a care label reading:*

*DELICATE. NO HARSH SHAMPOOS.
NO MACHINE-DRYING. AIR-DRY
ONLY. NEVER IRON.*

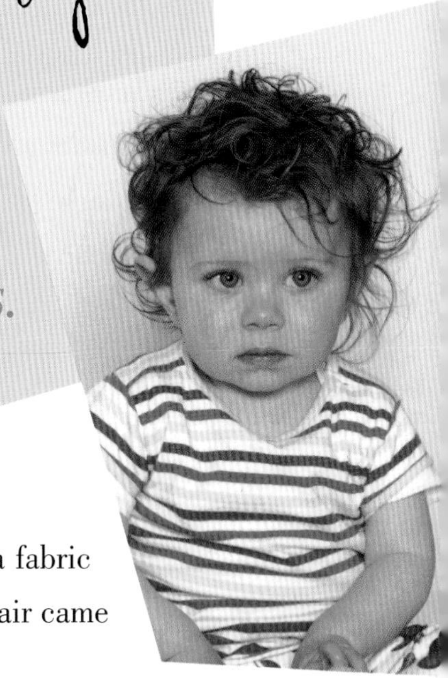

I love care labels in clothes. They make me respect a fabric and think carefully about how I treat it. If only our hair came with a care label.

All Hair Is Fiber

There isn't much difference chemically between your hair and the fine wool that comes off a pashmina goat. The one hundred thousand or so hair fibers on your head stretch and absorb moisture, just like wool, which is composed of the same elements as hair: carbon, hydrogen, nitrogen, oxygen, and sulfur. Because hair is a fiber, it makes sense to treat it like one. How do you care for the precious fibers in your wardrobe? You should handle your hair as gently as you do your cashmere sweater.

You'd never dream of washing a good sweater with detergent. Yet most shampoos contain harsh detergents (sodium lauryl sulfate or laureth sulfate) that one finds in dishwashing liquid. They're great for pots and pans because they cut grease so effectively. Your hair, on the other hand, needs to retain some natural oils, which protect it and your scalp. Stripping them away deprives the hair of necessary moisture and amino acids and makes it look dry and dull.

I'd like you to try this simple experiment to see what detergent does to your hair. Go into your kitchen and pour a bit of dishwashing detergent onto a damp sponge and squeeze gently. Voila, bubbles! Now, hold the sponge under running water and notice that it seems to take forever to rinse it free of the lather. You never really get rid of all that detergent, do you?

Your curls react the same way to shampoo: because curly hair is so porous, it absorbs detergent like a sponge. The truth is that lathers don't cleanse at all—manufacturers put lathering agents into products so you'll buy into the joy-of-suds myth. You know, those women in TV commercials moaning in ecstasy as they lather up their heads in the shower, then reappear seconds later with wonderfully styled hair, shining with vitality. Well, forget the

Hair Facts

Hair grows at a rate of about a half inch a month. It develops under your scalp, in a tiny sac called the follicle. Inside the follicle it's alive. When the hair comes to the surface the fiber hardens. The follicle will keep growing the hair for three to five years. When it stops growing, it goes into a period of rest—a few weeks only while the root is released from the follicle—then drops out. You lose about a hundred hairs a day, not a bad percentage considering you have at least one hundred thousand on your head at any given time. Within days after a hair is shed, another hair starts growing to replace it.

advertising campaigns that put sudsiness right up there next to cleanliness, god-liness, and sexiness. It doesn't work that way, and you don't have to buy into it.

I can't say this too often: *You do not need to use shampoo.* I'm not saying leave your hair dirty. As you read on, you'll see that I recommend cleansing the hair with . . . water and conditioner! My care routine for curly and wavy hair either cuts out shampoo entirely or cuts it down severely from your normal use. Whichever type of curly girl you are (see chapter 3), you're going to have to get out of the lather habit and end shampoo dependency—that ingrained belief that you have to wash your hair daily.

The Cuticle Is Critical

If you examine a cross section of a hair fiber under a microscope, you'll see that it looks like a worm. Growing around the worm's core are tiny scales, which cover the cortex or center of the hair like tiles on a roof. Those overlapping "tiles" are called the cuticle of the hair—and they're essential in protecting each strand and making your hair look good.

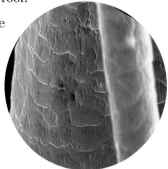

When the tiles lie flat, they reflect light and your hair shines. If the cuticle is ruffled, your hair won't shine because light needs to be reflected off a smooth surface. Detergents, heat, chemicals, or a hairbrush make the cuticle rough and scaly. Instead of lying flat, pieces of cuticle stick out and lock together like

A strand of healthy hair: the tile-like cuticles lie flat.

Velcro. So if you are using a blow-dryer to style your hair, stop, right now.

Lorraine's Shampoo Epiphany

In the bad old days, I would subject my scalp and hair to a vigorous lathering once or twice a week, for no good reason except force of habit. Afterward, for the first twenty-four hours, my hair would appear to float in space like a helium balloon, defying the laws of gravity, because I had ruffled the surface cuticle and dehydrated the curls. Another three days would go by before my hair had recovered enough from its trauma that I was ready to admit we were related. Then we'd happily coexist for the rest of the week, until it was time—according to my self-imposed regimen—for my next shampoo. And the vicious cycle would begin all over again.

I followed this routine unquestioningly, because I'd never found any care instructions that addressed the specific needs of curly, as opposed to straight, hair. Then one fateful morning I looked in the mirror and realized my hair looked fabulous. According to my schedule, I was due for a shampoo, but I couldn't bear to mess with success. I dared myself to wait another day. One stretched into a second, then a third, until I'd managed to hold out for almost three weeks. My hair had never looked better, so I decided to initiate an experiment: I would declare my hair a shampoo-free zone and see how long I could refrain from washing it with detergent.

Now shampoo is a total no-no in my home. I don't use it at all anymore, not even a drop. I work up a sweat running most mornings, I eat in smoky European restaurants, and I swim in the ocean not far from my home. Yet my friends assure me that I pass the sniff test. My hair and scalp don't smell—and my hair has never looked better.

The high heat damages the cuticle. And if you still iron your curls to straighten them (not likely since that was a seventies fad), you're destroying precious fibers with the heat.

Why Curly Hair
Is Drier

Most of us treat our hair and scalp as a single entity. But the scalp is very different from the hair. The hair is keratin; the scalp is skin and needs to be treated the way we treat our facial skin—by cleansing it gently and keeping it moisturized. Nature designs it that way: each hair follicle that produces the hair on our heads is also home to sebaceous (oil) glands, which release sebum, an oily substance that lubricates the hair. "Curly hair is so much dryer than other types of hair," says Dr. David H. Kingsley of the Institute of Trichologists, "because there are only about 100,000 hairs on a curly head, as opposed to about 120,000 straight hairs. And because there is less hair, there are fewer follicles and therefore fewer sebaceous glands to produce oil." If you have tight curly hair, the sebum sometimes has trouble getting to the ends, which tend to be especially dry. Those with corkscrew curls have to compensate with extra moisteners (see chapter 4) to replace the moisture that isn't getting to the ends.

It's possible to have dry hair and an oily scalp. Having combination skin (oily in the T-zone, but dry everywhere else) is one clue that you might have an oily scalp. The sebum and sweat, which your scalp produces, are sterile and clean, but they attract dirt and bacteria. These must be rinsed off regularly to keep the scalp healthy. But it's not necessary to remove all of the oils from your scalp; in fact, it's not healthy. You need a fine layer of sebum—called the acid mantle—to protect the scalp. My solution is to rinse the scalp daily, giving it a gentle rub and a good water rinsing. No harsh detergent is necessary.

It's in the Genes

If you look at a cross section of a strand of Asian hair (straight), you'll see that the shape of the fiber is round. (Think of toothpaste coming out of a tube.) A strand of curly hair, looked at in cross section, looks elliptical, with a slight curve in the middle (like ribbon candy). The center indentation makes it flex and spiral—in other words, curl. A strand of African American hair is flatter still than a strand of corkscrew curls, has the finest texture, and is therefore also the curliest. Wavy hair, on the other hand, looks oval under a microscope. Its spiral is gentler, and it bends very slightly. Your genetic inheritance determines whether your hair will be curly or straight.

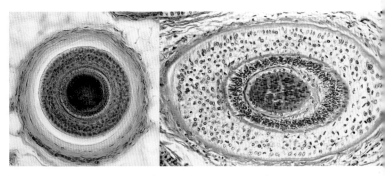

The fiber of straight hair (left) is round; a strand of wavy hair (right) is oval.

As a rule, curly hair is very fine and straight hair is coarse and stronger. Someone with tight curly corkscrews may appear to have thick hair because it has such volume. That's an optical illusion. The spirals fill more space and create the impression of texture. Pull a strand of that hair out to its full length and it will be fine and very fragile.

The morning of my father's funeral, I had a really bad hair day. I don't mean to sound disrespectful, but this was my worst nightmare come true. All my life, I'd suffered because of my curly hair: bad cuts, ill-fated attempts to grow my hair long, hours spent straightening it with hideous-smelling chemicals, dates gone bad because my hair had morphed into a giant ball of frizz. Not to mention all the nights when I slept (or tried to) with my curls tightly twisted around giant orange juice cans.

I was a short, timid, skinny kid who entered a new school in the middle of ninth grade on a rainy day when my hair did everything it shouldn't have. Thirty-eight years later, I still believe I would have had a socially successful high school career if only the sun had been shining and the humidity low as I walked into my first class. Worst of all were the Saturday mornings of my adolescence, most of which I spent in synagogue. My father was a rabbi, and I was expected to attend services every week. I would stand in front of the mirror, wailing because my hair had taken

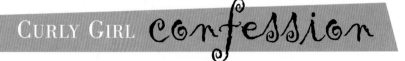

Hair straightened with orange juice cans

on shapes not known in nature. But my father refused to accept the frizz factor as a reason not to show up at services. I sat in synagogue week after week, hating my hair, myself, my life. I was convinced that I was the object of the entire congregation's collective pity and scorn. **I didn't have a bad hair day. I had a bad hair decade.**

After college, I became a school librarian. What better choice for a shy, bespectacled introvert who hated to be seen in public when the humidity was high? I started therapy, almost a residency requirement for the New York City neighborhood where I lived, and rehashed my childhood. I talked about how much misery my curls had caused me, especially as a teenager. **My therapist seemed to think that my unhappiness was related to other, more profound issues, but what did she know? Her hair was stick straight.**

Years passed. I quit my librarian job and went into publishing. I had my ears pierced, exchanged my glasses for contact lenses, began to emerge from my curl-related shell. Then came my father's unexpected death from a heart attack. On this most painful occasion of my life, when hundreds of people were expected to attend the funeral, I was furious because, once again, my hair had betrayed me. No doubt much of my reaction was misplaced grief, but my anticurl emotions ran deep and had a powerful hold over my psyche.

My story has a happy ending. I eventually met Lorraine, who encouraged me to stop fighting with my hair and cultivate my curls by growing them long. These days, I feel sexier, freer, more flirtatious, drawn to glitter and sequins. I am constantly astonished and gratified by my curls and people's reactions to them. My hair cascades down below my shoulders (and much farther when it's wet) in an explosion of corkscrews of varying lengths and textures. The curls change according to the dictates of the weather, and I love their many moods and shapes. They're easy to care for, now that I've given up trying to control them, and I never agonize about how my hair will look for a special event. I understand that as long as I treat my curls with respect (i.e., keep them well hydrated and properly nourished) and resist the urge to shampoo, blow-dry, or fuss, they won't ever embarrass me.

My hair gets lots of attention, which means I do, too, even more so as I experiment with different shades of color and highlights, depending on my mood and the season. Here's what I find most remarkable: I've become outgoing and friendly, a wallflower transformed into Miss Congeniality. I've discovered that basking in the limelight can be an emotionally uplifting experience. But having great curly hair is not without its responsibilities. I am frequently approached by curly girls hungry for information and moral support. **"If I can learn to be proud of my curls, so can you,"** I assure them, fulfilling my commitment to what Lorraine calls the curly girl mentoring program.

I've also had to revamp my wardrobe. A head of bouncy curls deserves better than T-shirts, khaki pants, navy blue blazers, and clogs. The safe, conservative outfits in my closet have been replaced by hip, free-spirited (or wild, depending on your point of view) clothes that are fun to wear and make me feel young. People tell me I look younger than I did before I became so well informed about what my curls need to stay happy. I think it's "psycurlogical," a perfect example of curly girl mind-body unity.

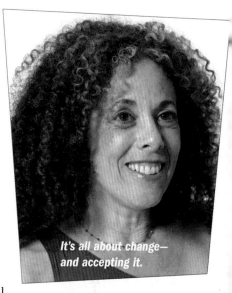

It's all about change—and accepting it.

Years ago, I found a card that showed a picture of Frieda, the redheaded, curl-obsessed *Peanuts* character, along with this wise-beyond-her-years statement: **People always expect more when you have naturally curly hair.** Now, finally, I am at one with Frieda. I have liberated my inner curl and let my spirit soar. I can meet any challenge. I am Curly Girl.

—DEBORAH CHIEL, WRITER

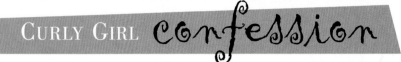
I would never have become a comedian if I'd been born with straight hair. Comedians need to have obstacles, and, boy, did I have them. Curls made my career. As I say in my book, "People who are successful take the good and build on it. I take the bad and build on that." It's what got me started in comedy clubs; all that anger motivated me. When I was growing up, I was the only one in my neighborhood stuck with curly hair. **People used to call me Brillo head.** They thought they were being original.

When I was really small, my mother used to brush out the knots in my hair with a wire brush that's normally used for grooming dogs. I screamed so much that she finally took me to a hairdresser at Best & Company on Fifth Avenue who had also worked on a curly-haired Italian princess in Italy. He cut my hair so short that it sat on my head like some sort of cactus. Not much different from a Brillo pad, actually.

In high school, I'd straighten my hair with chemicals so strong that I called them Agent Orange. It was the sixties and everybody then had to have "swinging hair." Kenneth, the hairdresser, became famous for giving people like Jackie Kennedy swinging hair. My hair does not swing. It springs. Or maybe it hops. On bad days it sinks.

In the seventies, I read that coffee separated curls and gave them weight. I'd brew coffee, wait until it was cold, then pour it over my head. My curls sagged, I looked awful, and I smelled of coffee. When I started doing stand-up comedy, I talked about how the hairdresser would pull my hair over giant rollers and spritz it with a ton of spray, so I'd look like an eighteenth-century composer. There I was, Beethoven with caffeine curves.

Now you should see how hard my hairdresser at *The View* has to work before a show. Everyone's afraid of curly hair on TV, because the light doesn't bounce off curls properly, or so they tell me. I think society needs to change its idea of what's pretty, but, personally, I still think I look better with straight hair. So sue me.

—**JOY BEHAR, COMEDIAN AND CO-HOST OF *THE VIEW***

My hair does not swing. It springs. Or maybe it hops.

Before I go on The View, everyone works hard to straighten my hair.

Chapter Three

THE THREE TYPES OF CURLY GIRLS

Which Curl Are You?

Curls are like snowflakes or fingerprints. No two are alike, making it difficult to generalize about curly hair. Some of us are born with tight corkscrew curls so relentless that not even Superman could stretch them out, so brittle that they break with the least resistance. Some of us have soft Botticelli curls that frame our faces with ringlets, making us look like angels in Renaissance paintings. And millions of us have varying degrees of curls and waves. Many of us fight them, straightening our hair with blow-dryers and rollers. In fact, some of us don't even know what our wave potential is. (See "Are You a Curly Girl?" on page 7.)

In order for you to know how to care for your particular curls or learn how to develop some waves, I've identified three types of curly girls—Corkscrew, Botticelli, and Wavy. For each type, I've used recognizable celebrities as identifying icons. Decide which celebrity and characteristics best match your hair, then go straight to the particular care routine for your "curl type" (see chapter 4) to learn how to nurture and encourage those curls.

CORKSCREW

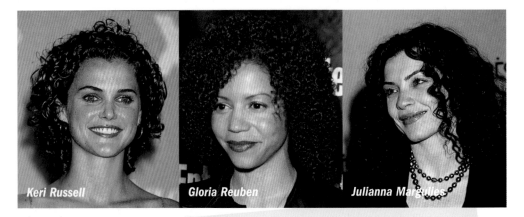

Keri Russell Gloria Reuben Julianna Margulies

YOU KNOW YOU HAVE CORKSCREW HAIR IF YOU HAVE:

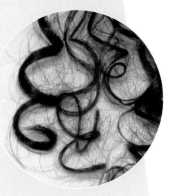

☐ Curls as tightly wound as a French poodle's if cut too short

☐ Lots of small coils of curls

☐ Superdry hair that crackles with electricity

☐ A high frizz factor

☐ Very dry skin

☐ Curls that tend to stand out from your head instead of lying flat

☐ Hair that soaks up as much conditioner as you feed it

Many Corkscrew divas believe their hair is thickly textured, but separate a single strand and you'll discover that it is actually baby fine and very delicate. That's why it breaks so easily, as African Americans can testify (see chapter 6). And because the cuticle stands out instead of lying flat, the curls catch and the hair snarls easily. Most tangles and snarls are found under the top layer of hair, at the nape of the neck.

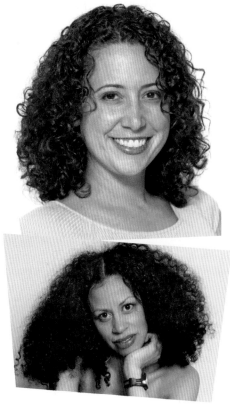

Because Corkscrew curls are so very dry, your mantra should be moisturize, moisturize, moisturize. Hydrate your scalp as often as you apply moisturizer to your face and give your curls lots of TLC as you follow the care routine in chapter 4. African American curly hair is most similar to Corkscrew curls in fragility and dryness. But because it has special needs, I've dealt with it in a separate chapter.

If you follow the care routine on pages 30–38, you can have glorious Corkscrew curls that live up to their potential:

- Well-hydrated curls with spring and shine
- Low frizz factor, even in humid weather
- Short hair that keeps its shape
- Long hair with well-defined ringlets

BOTTICELLI CURLS

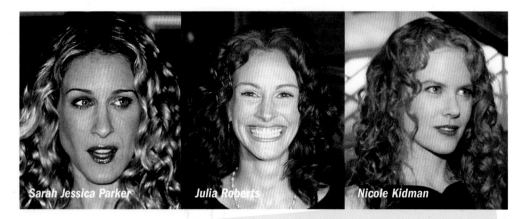

Sarah Jessica Parker

Julia Roberts

Nicole Kidman

YOU KNOW YOU HAVE BOTTICELLI HAIR
IF YOU HAVE:

☐ Curls that vary in size

☐ Curls that fall gracefully down your head instead
of sticking straight out

☐ Texture that is medium-fine

☐ Hair that is brittle and easily damaged

☐ Curls that sometimes cannot be coaxed into
making an appearance because they're weighed
down by the top layer of hair

Like people with tight curls, Botticelli curly girls have to keep their hair well hydrated with humectants and emollients (see chapter 5), but this kind of hair needs less conditioner for its daily routine. The curls are looser, in the shape of soft *S*'s. Follow the directions that begin on page 30 for Corkscrew and Botticelli curls, noting the differences in amounts of conditioner and how often you can rinse your hair. Once your hair has regained the necessary moisture (it takes two to three weeks), you'll probably be able to cut back on the conditioner.

Botticelli girls who want to live up to their name can have:

- Soft, cascading curls that look wonderful long or short
- Hair that can be worn in a variety of styles
- Hair that is very forgiving
- Well-defined curls released from beneath the top layer, or canopy

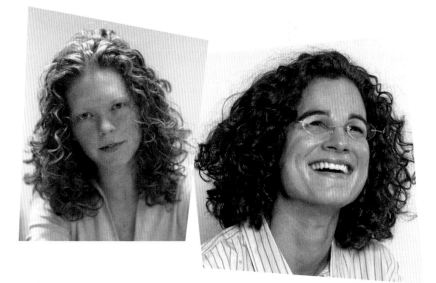

WAVY CURLS

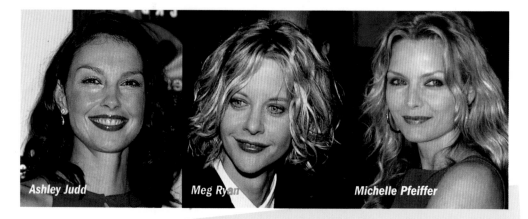

Ashley Judd

Meg Ryan

Michelle Pfeiffer

YOU KNOW YOU HAVE WAVY HAIR IF YOU HAVE:

☐ Hair that you've always believed was straight

☐ Hair that on humid days is surrounded by a halo of frizz

☐ Hair that occasionally develops a natural wave, which you've tried to blow-dry out

☐ Hair that has a tendency to look unkempt

☐ Hair that is flat on the crown

☐ Had wavy hair when you were very young

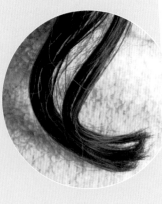

I estimate that 65 percent of all women have wavy or curly hair, but many have never been aware of it or have been fighting their natural bent and misunderstanding their hair for years. Many of the women who fall into this huge category frequently wear their hair completely straight. The kinds of waves also vary greatly, even on the same head of hair. Some wavy hair can have a curl spring factor of five inches, while other wavy curls fall in extremely lazy *S*'s below the shoulders. Those wavy girls who think they are straight may be on too strict a haircut schedule, so that the waves are cut before they have a chance to develop. It's important to let wavy hair grow to its best length—giving the entire *S*-wave a chance to grow out. (See chapter 7.)

If you're a Wavy type and have always worn your hair straight and short, you may want to try to realize your curl potential. Check the characteristics on the facing page. Follow the directions on pages 40–44 for three weeks and you may be surprised to discover you're a curly girl, too. Treat your hair gently and bring out its full wavy potential:

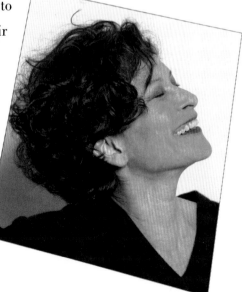

- Loose, glamorous curls that need a minimum care routine
- Hair that is very versatile, whether short finger waves or an updated Farrah Fawcett look
- Wavy hair that shines with good health

Curly Cue: The Spring Factor

The tightness of your curls (or spring factor) is a sure way to determine which type of curly girl you are. It's something your hairdresser should know or be told because it tells him or her how much to cut. Basically, the spring factor is the difference in the length of a curl when it falls naturally and when it's extended. Here's how to check yours: Pull a strand of dry curls down against your shoulder or neck to its full length. Leave your finger at the point where the strand touches. Now let go. With a ruler, measure the distance between your finger and where your curl naturally ends. The number is your personal spring factor. It will help you determine which hair-care routine to follow.

9- to 12-inch spring = Corkscrew curls

5- to 8-inch spring = Botticelli curls

2- to 4-inch spring = Wavy curls

If you have short hair, your spring factor would be about half as long as the figures above.

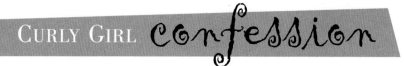

My first—and worst—hair trauma occurred when I was nine. I had very long, curly hair that fell halfway down my back, and I loved wearing it loose and carefree. My parents, who thought my hair looked unruly, announced that if I didn't start taking care of it, I'd have to get it cut off. One day, in the dead of winter, my mother made good on her threat and dragged me to a beauty parlor to get my hair cut in a short shag. I was so humiliated by the result that I decided to wear a knit cap to school until my hair grew back.

Don't even ask me what I went through in high school. It was the late seventies, when everyone but me had straight Farrah Fawcett hair. (I wonder if she has any idea how many curly girls suffered because of her hairstyle.) I'd wash my hair every night, blow it dry straight, and pull it back in a pony-tail. Then I'd wake up at 6:00 A.M. and wrap it around hot rollers to complete the treatment. The day of my senior prom, I was even more obsessed than usual with the weather report. We lived in Pittsburgh, Pennsylvania, where it is very humid, and the May mist is a nightmare. I was wearing a to-die-for, off-the-shoulder gown, and I wanted my hair to be equally sleek. When I woke up that morning, the weather was hot and humid, and as the hours passed, the air remained laden with moisture. I gave up and let my hair do its thing.

When I emerged from my bedroom, my mother looked stunned. "Your hair looks beautiful," she said. "That's how you should always wear it." I was horrified.

I'd imagined myself as Farrah Fawcett, and I'd morphed into Shirley Temple.

When we arrived at the prom, I locked eyes across the ballroom with Mark, the boy I'd had a crush on since fourth grade. Like a scene from a movie, we walked toward each other, meeting halfway. "You look so beauti-ful," he said. "I can't believe what your hair looks like." We kissed passionately, right there in front of our dates. It was a magical moment. Then he threw up all over his shoes. He was totally wasted.

But he loved my hair.

—**SHELLEY OZKAN,**
FULL-TIME MOTHER

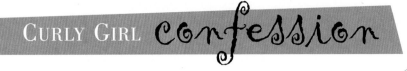
The Curly Life

Curls are so much more than just responsive little ringlets. They move, they breathe, they have attitude, they take positions. Curls embody all the qualities of freedom and fun that stir up our lives and stimulate our imaginations. In their resilience, in their ability to bounce back and find their own form, curls invent themselves over and over again.

You might even say (I have said it) that curls are revolutionary. They resist everything but their own impulses. Curls twist like Möbius strips, flex like flying fish, swerve like the circuitry in silicon chips, rise up like waveforms, and crackle like well-fed fires.

A curly girl is always a curly girl, even when her curls are hiding. My own curls were incognito for years, subdued by barrettes, braids, bobby pins, bows, sprays, and serious brushings. But curls are a Force of Nature and one wet summer Nature herself came down in a series of storms that transformed my strained and straightened hair into a cloud of cumulous curls.

I could hate my curls or I could love them, but I couldn't do anything about them. I decided not to hate them. It was like the first principle of riding a roller coaster: **Accept the curve, be delighted, and never look back.**

BY JOAN SCHENKAR

Chapter Four

THE CURLY GIRL PROGRAM

Creating a Daily Routine

The program of daily hair care that's mapped out in this chapter is truly revolutionary. Adopting it means you'll have to give up a lot of assumptions you have about what constitutes good hair grooming. But if you've lived with curly hair all your life and put up with frizz, parched curls, and horrendous bad hair days, you're probably ready to start. I guarantee it will change your life.

Some of you—those I've classified as "Wavy" (see chapter 3)—will have to cut back on how often you shampoo your hair. But most curly girls will have to do something extraordinary—throw out every bottle of shampoo in the bathroom and get rid of your blow-dryer!

I'm going to show you how to keep your hair and scalp clean using only water and conditioner. Yes, conditioner. Once you break your shampoo dependency, you'll still be rinsing your hair daily, but in a way that will keep it shiny and healthy, instead of constantly stripping it of lubrication with the harsh detergents found in most shampoos. And you'll be letting your hair air-dry as well.

DAILY ROUTINE
FOR CORKSCREW AND
BOTTICELLI CURLS

Cleansing

Your daily curly hair routine starts every morning in the shower. (If you decide to skip a shower one morning, simply spritz, scrunch, and go. See "Curls on the Go," page 45.) About once a week, cleanse your hair and scalp with conditioner, as in step 2 (below). On other days, after wetting your hair thoroughly, go to step 3. While you wean yourself off shampoo, you may want to use conditioner to cleanse your hair twice a week. After that, once a week or every ten days is enough.

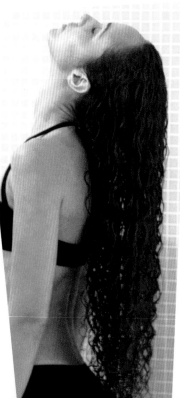

1 Step under the shower as if you're standing under a waterfall or are caught in a sudden cloudburst. (The pressure can be moderately heavy.) Don't touch your hair yet. Let the water cascade through your curls in the way they fall naturally. Resist the impulse to start scrubbing your head and disarranging your hair's basic shape.

2 Take a half teaspoon of conditioner. It can be a regular or a leave-in conditioner, as long as it's rich in emollients and humectants. (See chapter 5.) With your fingertips and this bit of conditioner you're going to cleanse your scalp, loosening any residue that's accumulated. Believe me, the conditioner and the stimulation from your fingers will work as well as shampoo. Starting at the temples, rub gently down the sides, then move to the

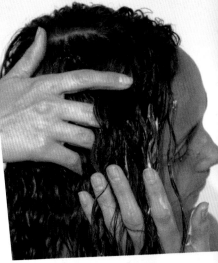

top of your head, scrubbing gently toward the crown. Finally, move down the back of your head, finishing up at the nape. Now let the shower spray wash through your entire head, rinsing out whatever your fingers have loosened. Your scalp is clean now. Still worried about sweat and other buildup? Remember that sweat and sebum are sterile. But they do attract bacteria if left too long. However, friction is a time-tested method of cleaning (think of a washing machine churning), and it will remove everything that needs to be removed without harming your hair or scalp.

How Much Conditioner?

In general, the tighter or dryer the curl, the more conditioner you need. I suggest average amounts of conditioner here, but you are going to have to monitor usage on the basis of your hair's needs. If your hair has been damaged by coloring or too much blow-drying and chemical straightening, it probably absorbs conditioner very fast and will need more. You'll have to experiment with what amount of conditioner is best for your hair. If you apply too much conditioner, the worst that can happen is your hair will look overcoated and dull that day. Not a bad trade-off, considering you're making your hair healthier and shinier in the long run.

3 Now rub a half teaspoon of conditioner (a blob about the size of a quarter) between your hands and smooth the conditioner on the outer layer (or canopy) of your hair—the part that is most exposed to the elements. Work another half teaspoon under the hair at the nape of your neck, the spot most prone to tangles and knots. Be gentle because the hair there breaks easily. Using your fingers as a comb, gently comb through your hair from underneath, removing any loose hairs. Don't get nervous. Remember, it's normal to lose about a hundred hairs a day!

4 Spread another half teaspoon of conditioner through the hair at each side of your head, using your fingers as a comb. (Botticelli types may find that this is too much and weighs down their curls.) The point is to distribute the

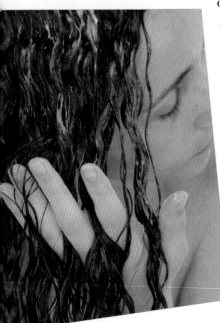

conditioner evenly through your curls so they don't fuse with each other, which, as you now know, can damage the cuticle.

Your hair should feel smooth and silky right now—almost like wet seaweed. Over time, you'll know instinctively whether or not to rinse out the conditioner at this point. If you do rinse, just let the shower spray fall over your head for a few seconds to evenly distribute the conditioner without removing all of it.

Bonus: At this point, you can rinse your hair just a little more and give it a wonderful lavender scent by spritzing your curls with some homemade Lavender Mist. (See "Lorraine's Lotions and Potions," page 53.) Comb it through with your fingers.

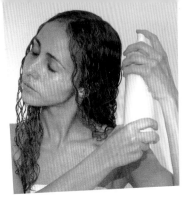

Spot-Cleaning

Just as you may clean a spot on a blouse, where perhaps you spilled red wine, you may occasionally want to spot-clean your scalp. If your scalp feels itchy or oily in one or two patches, put a dab of conditioner on your fingertips and scrub directly on the spot. Then rinse thoroughly. If you are still using shampoo, first coat the ends of your hair with conditioner, then spot-wash with shampoo. The spot-cleaning technique applies to all types of curly hair—Corkscrew, African American, Botticelli, and Wavy.

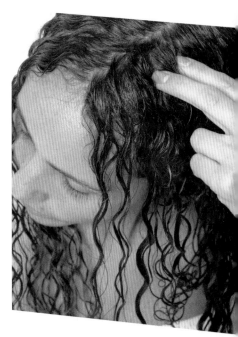

Drying

1 Step out of the shower and grab a hand towel. Bend forward and cup your hair loosely in the towel, then scrunch it upward toward the scalp to blot up the moisture. Do not wring or rub it dry.

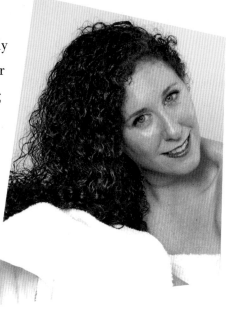

2 Beginning at the back of the head, gently squeeze sections of hair. Continue all around your head, blotting any sections that are still dripping wet. Do it gently, going with the natural waves and without disturbing the hair too much. Remember the sweater analogy—after washing, you blot it dry in a towel so as not to disturb the fibers. And by now you know your hair is a precious fiber. Rotate the towel occasionally so that one section doesn't get sopping wet and lose its absorbency.

Styling and Air-Drying

Remember curly girl rule number one: Resist the temptation to blow-dry your hair at this point. Your curls need to recover their shape, not get blown out of proportion.

1 Take a tablespoon of a clear styling gel (see chapter 5) and rub it into your palms. Bend over to let your curls fall free. Starting at the ends, scrunch the gel in toward the scalp. I call this motion the accordion technique. As you are doing it, visualize the undulating waves and folds of an accordion as a slow tune is played on it. Start scrunching at the nape and work

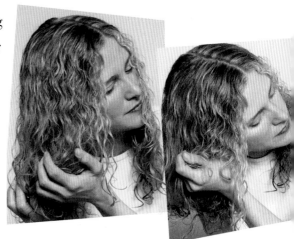

around your head, scrunching the top layer (canopy) of your hair last.

2 Now it's time to have some fun—and shape your curls. Go to the mirror. Scrunch sections of curls with your palms, pushing up and squeezing gently into place. For shorter or looser curls, twist the hair around a finger and clip. Or put a bit of gel directly on a clip before fastening it. This will help hold the front curls and give a little lift at the top.

Remember, your hair is still drying, so wherever you place your curls now, that's how they'll dry. Take another half teaspoon of gel and, ever so gently, graze your hands over the top layer of hair (don't be heavy-handed). This will minimize frizz.

3 To get the curls on the top of your head to stand a little taller, you need to lift and clip the hair at the roots. This method releases the top layer of hair from its own weight and allows it to dry faster.

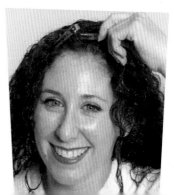

Using a clawlike motion, lift a small amount of hair from the top of your head. (Hair should be pulled perpendicular to the scalp, neither forward nor back-

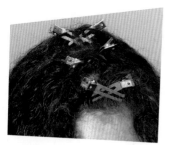

ward.) Place a clip at the roots where you pinched it and at right angles to the scalp. Make sure it's as tight as when you pinched it. Secure with a second clip (left). As a rule, you will need about six clips to "lift" the top of your hairdo—in front, at the crown, and between these two points.

If you want to disguise a part, take strands from either side and cross them over the part (right), then pin two curls on either side of it.

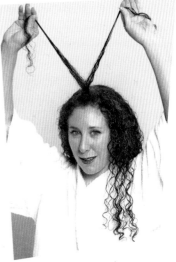

Once you've pinned everything you want lifted, leave your hair alone. Don't touch it for an hour. Let it dry, have some breakfast, get dressed, read the paper. Whatever you do, don't interrupt the curls or they'll frizz up. Remember, if you like the way your hair looks wet, you'll like how it looks when it dries.

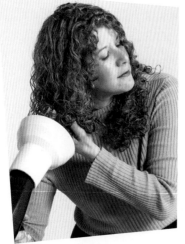

If you don't have time to air-dry your hair, dry it with a diffuser (a shallow, bowl-shaped attachment that reduces the volume of air flow). You can control the effects of the diffuser by cupping your hand and lifting the section of hair that you're drying, so that the top layer of curls isn't blown every which way. To cut back on heat

Lorraine's Geography Lesson

We curly girls are natural weather barometers. Any increase in humidity, the slightest hint of rain or mist, and our hair gets big. I call this the east-west effect, hair that balloons out on either side of the head but lies flat on top, making you look a little like the Sphinx. (Think Gilda Radner's Roseanne Roseannadanna in *Saturday Night Live*.) Not a good look.

You need to train the curls on the top of your head to stand taller, so that your hair moves in a north-south direction as well. The easiest way to create this effect is to

Roseannadanna's east-west effect

use what I call the Playtex bra technique because it *lifts and separates* the top layer of curls. Follow step 3 (see page 35), which explains how to use clips to lift your hair at the roots after you wash it. Then hang a "Do Not Disturb" sign for yourself on your head and don't touch it during the drying process.

Note: Well-informed curly girls—those who have healthy hair and a pro-curl attitude—often opt for a style that moves in a more east-west direction. You, too, may decide, once you get comfortable with your curls, to push your boundaries and be more daring. For a wilder, sexier look, place your fingers an inch or two above the roots on either side of your head and shake gently. You'll expand your hair in an east-west direction without sacrificing control or style.

Weekly Scalp Treatment
(for All Hair Types)

We know that exfoliating is good for improving the condition of your skin. Since your scalp is also skin, give it a special exfoliating treatment once a week or so. Exfoliating will slough off any dead skin cells or conditioner buildup, making your scalp healthier and relieving any itchiness. Mix up and apply the Exfoliating Scrub (below).

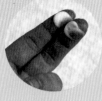

EXFOLIATING SCRUB

1 tablespoon brown sugar or quinoa (available at health food stores)
3 tablespoons conditioner

1. Mix together to create a thick consistency.
2. Wet your hair in the shower, then rub the paste on your fingertips. Apply to scalp and massage gently in a circular motion, starting at the nape of your neck and moving upward. Linger on any spots that seem tense or itchy.
3. Rinse thoroughly, then condition.

exposure, use a travel dryer, because its airflow is slower and weaker.

When your hair is completely dry, remove the clips gently. Look in the mirror. Bend over and shake your head a little. With your fingers, gently fluff your hair from underneath. Don't touch the top layer. If you still don't have enough height to suit your taste, you can use bobby pins and pin the curls just as you did with the clips. Get bobby pins the same color as your hair and you can wear them outside or to work. No one will notice. That's a great thing about curly hair—it hides a lot of scalp.

Second chance: If anything looks out of place, now's the time to make a quick fix. Use a couple of spritzes of a spray gel. Lift the curls you want to be higher, clip them as above, and wait until they dry before removing pins. If some curls seem too tight, clip a pin on the ends for a few seconds to loosen the coil.

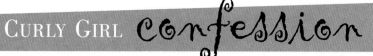

When I was a little girl, I was so desperate for straight hair that moved when I turned my head that I begged my mother to buy me a bathing cap with a ponytail attached to it. For a while, my mother had my hair cut very short—I suppose to make it more manageable—and people thought I was a boy, which of course I hated. When it was longer, she'd tie it back in two tight pigtails, like the ones Kathy wore on *Father Knows Best*.

As a teenager, I tried everything to banish the curls. I'd slather Dippity-Do styling gel on my hair, then tape it down. I don't know *where* I got this idea, but somehow it made sense. When I'd remove the tape in the morning, I'd often strip away pieces of skin with it. Because I'm short and small-boned, I always thought I looked better with my hair up and away from my face. I wore it in a French braid for several years—until I threw my back out braiding.

Whenever I went to a hair salon, I'd get very uptight because I would always have to tell the stylist what to do with my curls. She didn't have a clue. I would insist that she leave it long enough to "put it back in a ponytail."

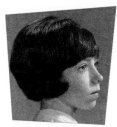

Curls banished with Scotch tape.

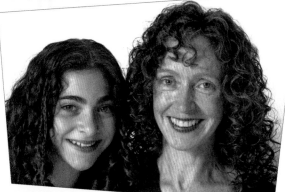

Patti and daughter, Dena, who loves her curls.

Then Dena entered my life. At age two my daughter would cry in front of the mirror whenever she looked at her mop of dark ringlets. She'd also clip handkerchiefs to the sides of her head to pretend she had long, straight hair. I worried that maybe she was learning this from me, and I began to wear my hair in curls—and not always tied back. Now that Dena is a teenager, she wears her hair long and curly.

It took me until my late forties to accept my curls. The fact remains that my hair will always be something to contend with. Given a choice, I'd still prefer straight hair that I could wear simple and short; it'd make my life and job easier—I own my own custom-made cookie company, so I always have to keep my hair tied back. But, for the first time in my life, I don't hide my ringlets.

—PATTI PAIGE,
OWNER OF BAKED IDEAS

DAILY ROUTINE FOR WAVY HAIR

Where there's a wave, there's a curl; that's my motto. This routine is meant to get wavy hair into great shape (with extra hydration) and to encourage the memory of its natural curl.

Wavy hair lies flat against the scalp but has gentle *S* waves. It can be coarse or fine and the strength of the waves varies greatly. If you have this kind of hair, you've probably been blow-drying it straight. If your hair is short, the curl may not even be discernible. Every curl is in the shape of an *S*. Some are very loose, floppy *S*'s. You have to let your hair grow into the length of the second part of the *S* before it springs into place naturally. Sometimes the hair has to grow past your shoulders before this happens.

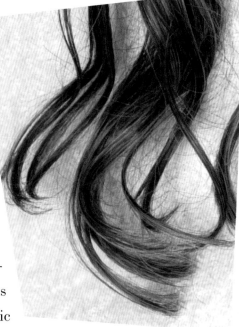

Wavy hair generally isn't as dry as really curly hair so you may choose to use shampoo— but only once a week. Check out the cosmetics and personal care section of your local organic or health food store for shampoos that contain little or no detergent. (See chapter 5.) The most radical changes for wavy hair are: when you shampoo your hair, always apply conditioner *first*. Stop using a blow-dryer to dry your hair straight. Never brush. Of course, if you get up and decide your hair doesn't need a complete wetting down, simply spritz with water, scrunch, and go. (See "Curls on the Go," page 45.)

Now, here's your basic wavy routine. On the days when you're not using shampoo, just follow steps 1 and 4.

Cleansing

1 Wet your hair under a gentle shower, letting the water simply flow through it. (You don't want to disturb any natural waves in your hair, so don't disarrange the basic shape of your hair while washing it.)

2 Now take a tablespoon of conditioner (see chapter 5) and, using your fingers, lightly coat your hair from the ends to the midshaft. This hair has been around longer than the hair at the roots and needs more lubrication. The conditioner protects the hair by not allowing shampoo to penetrate and dehydrate the shaft.

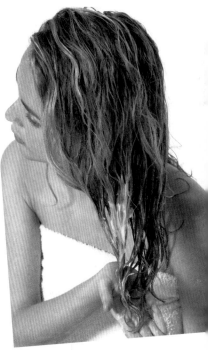

3 If you're using shampoo, squeeze a half teaspoon (no more) onto your fingertips and apply it gently to the scalp and roots only. Don't use your nails. Start at the forehead and work around the scalp. Then rinse thoroughly.

4 Add a half teaspoon of conditioner to your hair, and work it through with your fingers. Then rinse quickly, for just a few seconds. Now you're ready to blot-dry your hair.

Drying and Styling

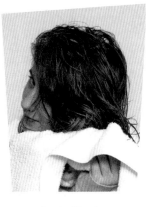

1 Cup a hand towel in your hands and bend forward. Scrunch your hair toward the scalp in an upward motion. Blot the hair to get rid of moisture, but don't twist or wring the hair dry. Start at the back and gently squeeze sections of hair. Continue all around the head, rotating the towel so no one section gets sopped.

2 Rub a tablespoon of styling gel (see chapter 5) on your palms. You're about to encourage any natural waves that you have. Bend forward, looking at the floor. Scrunch in the gel, starting at the back of the head, then the sides. With both hands, scrunch the hair on the top of your head; then straighten up, still holding the hank of hair. Let go and you'll see the natural waves in the canopy.

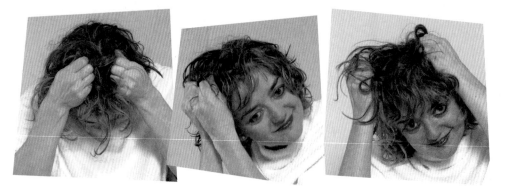

Encourage them with more scrunching—always from the end toward the scalp. Look in the mirror—the way your hair looks now when it's wet is how it will look dry.

3 To prevent a flat top, you'll need to lift and clip some curls on the crown of your head. This separates the curls so they dry faster. (See "Lorraine's Geography Lesson," page 37.) Short-haired Wavy girls can use four 1-inch clips, lifting and pinning two sections at the back of the crown, two nearer the forehead.

If your hair is long and thick, you may need a couple of butterfly clips to lift and hold the waves. Simply clasp a wave in the clip and close it.

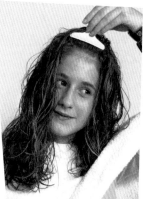

Playtex bra technique: lift and separate

4 Let your hair air-dry, if possible. If you're in a hurry, you can dry your hair with a diffuser. Instead of blasting your hair with a single stream of hot air, which can damage the cuticle and make the hair frizzy, you dry it gently without disturbing the waves. (Set the temperature on low.) Cup individual sections of waves, scrunching them a little to encourage the curl, and then aim the diffuser just on that section. Work around the head from back to side, to top.

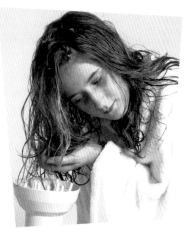

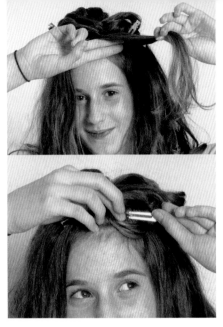

5 If you want a curlier look, try the pin curl method. Starting at the crown, wrap a section of hair around your finger, slide your finger out, hold the coil with your other hand, and insert a clip at right angles. (The pin curls should stand out from your head, not lie flat.) Do your entire head in giant pin curls. Air-dry or, if time is short, use a diffuser set on low. When your hair is dry, gently pull out the pins or clips and loosen your curls with your fingers.

Those of you who are not yet believers in your curls will have to practice this method on faith. I promise that within two or three weeks you will find your waves are well established. They've been waiting for you to treat them this way for years!

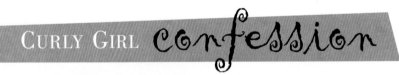

CURLY GIRL *confession*

My husband thinks my hair matches my character. Before our wedding, we wrote letters, saying why we wanted to marry each other. During the ceremony, the rabbi read an excerpt from my husband's letter: "The physical attributes that first hooked me on Rikki—her eyes, her smile, her hair—still continue to thrill me. Rikki's hair reflects her personality: at times wild and unruly, because Rikki is spontaneous and alive; at other times controlled and strong, because Rikki can also be focused and determined."

—RIKKI LANE, DOCTOR

Curls on the Go

If you wake up one morning and don't feel like showering or going through your usual hair care routine, use the Lavender Mist (see recipe on page 53) to refresh your curls quickly. Spray lightly—five or six spritzes at most—then take one curl at a time and twist it around your finger. Slide the hair off your finger and clip it horizontally at the root. The curls should be positioned around your head in soft

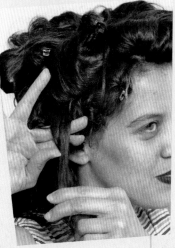

circles. For a quick fix, position about five curls on the crown of the head. If you have more time, use more. Let the curls dry for five to twenty minutes, then carefully remove the clips. Shake your head, loosen hair at scalp with fingers, admire your curls in the mirror, and go.

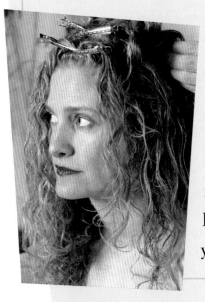

My hair is not curly; it has a wave to it. When I get out of the shower, and I let my hair air-dry, I have the most disgusting rat's nest on my head that anyone has ever seen. I used to have naturally wavy hair that turned into nice curls if I scrunched them and used lots of products. But I haven't trained it to be curly since I was sixteen.

For the last eleven years, I've been drying my hair straight to the point of destroying it. My hair is so brittle and won't grow past the middle of my back, because I'm always getting it cut. I use a hair dryer every day, even when I don't wash it, then I pin it up at night to keep it straight, so I don't wake up with knots in my hair.

I *know* I'm damaging it, but I'm insecure about it. **I know what I'm doing is terrible, but I still continue to straighten my hair.** I've learned to deal with all of my other body image issues, and I'm grateful for how I look. But my hair is the one thing left that I haven't accepted and I'd give anything to change.

—**BERTHA BRACKEN, ACTRESS AND STUDENT**

Before

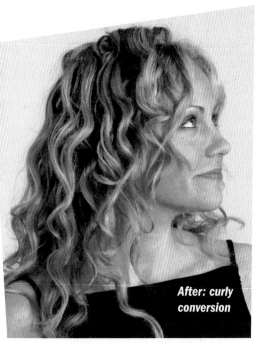

After: curly conversion

Chapter Five

PRODUCTS AND HOME REMEDIES

What's a Curly Girl to Do?

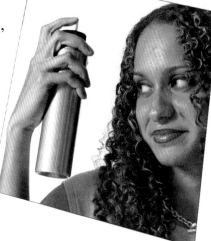

Curly girls tend to obsess about products, buying every new one that comes along in hopes of making their hair straighter, shinier, frizz-free, easier to manage. My care routine will get you out of that habit. *You'll need to buy only two products—a conditioner and a clear styling gel.* For Wavy types who will still shampoo their hair once in a while, I've suggested some alternatives to harsh shampoos.

I recently spent half an hour at one of my favorite beauty supply stores, checking out various brands of conditioners and gels. Here are some of the words I found on the packages: conditioning fixative, antifrizz lotion, texturizing creme, styling wax, forming gel, relaxing cream, moisturizing balm, hydrating cream, supporting liquid gel, nourishing cream, restorative cream, volume gel, moisturizing conditioner. Faced with all this jargon, what's a curly girl to do?

First, don't be fooled by the hype; if you read carefully, you'll see that many of the ingredients are identical from one brand to the next. But it's important to know what you're looking for in a product and how to read a label.

Talk to other women with hair similar to yours. Before buying, borrow or trade products with your curly-haired friends. Two or three uses should give you enough time to decide whether or not you like a particular conditioner or gel. If you've found a good stylist for curly hair, ask what she suggests for your hair. Hairdressers keep up with the latest advances in hair care products and experiment with different brands until they find two or three to recommend to clients. The information that follows is meant to help guide you through the product jungle, but ultimately you're the only one who can decide what keeps your curls happy and well nourished.

Shampoo

I've already talked about how harsh shampoos can damage your hair. The detergents seen most frequently on shampoo labels are sodium lauryl sulfate (the harshest), ammonium laureth sulfate (also harsh), and sodium laureth sulfate (a little gentler). Try to avoid products with the first two ingredients. It's best to water shampoos down with equal amounts of spring or distilled water or buy a product that lists plant extracts or buffering ingredients such as disodium EDTA or citric acid high up on the label.

What to Look for on a Label

Always look at shampoo labels before buying. As on a food label, ingredients are listed from most amount to least. Water is frequently the first ingredient, which means it's what you're spending most of your money on. Look for *cocamidopropyl betaine* on the label; it's the gentlest kind of cleaning agent and is found in baby shampoos. It doesn't lather as well, so it will not harm your hair as much as harsh detergents.

If you're shopping in a natural food store, look for *decyl polyglucose,* a natural cleaning agent, or shampoos made from olive oil or wheat germ oil.

You don't need shampoos with built-in conditioners. You're going to follow a different program, which involves applying conditioner to your hair before you shampoo, so that extra ingredient is unnecessary.

Conditioners

In general, leave-in conditioners don't contain enough emollients and humectants, so I generally don't recommend using them. However, as you'll see from my routine for Corkscrew curls, you will be leaving in a small amount of regular conditioner. Some curly girls, especially those who live in cold-weather regions, find that they need a thicker, richer conditioner during the winter months.

Reading the labels of conditioners can be confusing since so many ingredients just add to the thickness, fragrance, or look of the product itself and have no benefit for the hair. I suggest that you avoid conditioners with silicones. Although they do add temporary shine to the hair, I find they weigh down curly hair. (That means avoid using products with ingredients whose names end in *-cone.*) *The ingredients you absolutely need in a conditioner include emollients, humectants, proteins, and moisturizers.* Here's what to look for:

Emollients soften and smooth skin and reduce frizz in hair by smoothing the cuticle. There are hundreds of emollients. Shea butter is found in a lot in products for African American hair and it's excellent for most curly types. Others to look for include vegetable oils, wheat germ, olive and walnut oils.

Proteins coat the hair shaft and protect it. Look for plant proteins such as wheat, wheat germ, or soy protein on the back of the label.

Also, make sure your diet includes lots of protein because it's necessary for keeping your hair healthy from the inside out.

Humectants absorb water and hold in moisture. They are absolutely crucial in a conditioner for curly hair. Panthenol, vegetable glycerine, and sorbitol are just a few humectants to look for on the label.

Moisturizers add softness and control to curly hair. Amino acids and aloe vera are two great moisturizers.

Styling Gel

You don't need to know the chemical formula to buy a gel that's right for your curls, but here's what you do need to know. A clear gel is preferable; it's the last product you put into your hair before it dries, and you want your own color to shine through. (White or yellow-tinted gel can leave a film on the hair and, over time, make it look dull.) Look for a gel that doesn't contain alcohol and that has little or no fragrance. But it should contain the ingredients PVP (polyvinylpyrrolidone) and PVP/VA (vinyl acrylate).

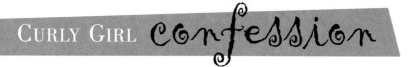

I am a twenty-seven-year-old curly girl desperately in need of help. It's been a grueling journey: bad hair days; poor self-image and low self-esteem; a cabinet full of gels, mousses, and chemical straightening products; years of wishing for "beautiful, straight hair."

I wash my hair every day and plan my life around it. If I have a date after work but want to go to the gym in the afternoon, I worry about when I'll have the time to wash my hair. Forget about spontaneous—anything! Often, I prefer not to go out after work because I don't like the way my hair looks.

I'm a slave to weather forecasts and have a long list of life events—junior prom, graduations, Florida vacations—ruined by my bad hair. When my brother got married this past June, I had my hair cut and styled in an updo right before the wedding. What a nightmare! It was one of the hottest days of the summer, and I hated how my hair looked. I couldn't stop crying. Even today, I could cry looking at the pictures, and it wasn't even my wedding!

My bathroom is a product graveyard. I'll try a twelve-dollar gel once and decide it doesn't work, so I'll stick it under the sink. The truth is, I'd spend any amount of money to fulfill my fantasy of having straight hair. I'm a new woman when I get my hair blown out. I can walk into any room and feel like a queen. But I usually don't have time for that, except on special occasions.

My last boyfriend was very sensitive to my negative feelings about my curly hair. He always complimented me and told me how much he liked it. I hope that I can find another man who understands that **dealing with my curls is a major part of my existence**.

I don't think people realize the struggles we curly-haired women endure.

—BROOKE HIRSCHFELDER, CORPORATE HUMAN RESOURCES ADMINISTRATOR

When shopping for gel, do the skin test: if it feels sticky on your skin, it will feel sticky on your hair. You also want to avoid styling creams and waxes because they can make your hair look crispy and petrified, like ramen noodles.

If your hair is thick and wavy, you may need to use more gel, but a light hold works best for curly girls with fine hair. Spray styling gels are basically diluted versions of gels. They're especially good on loose, wavy curls because the mist gets lightly distributed through the hair without weighing it down. They're also a wonderful way to refresh all hair types during the day. (See "Curls on the Go," page 45.)

You can even make your own spray gel by combining $1/2$ cup gel with 1 cup boiled water. Allow to cool, then pour into a spray bottle. If you think your hair needs a stronger hold, experiment by gradually adding more gel to the mixture until you achieve the consistency that works best for your curls.

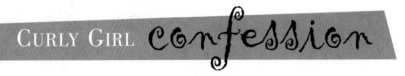

CURLY GIRL confession

I used to live in Washington, D.C., where a person's political affiliation is a typical ice-breaker at cocktail parties. At one gathering, a man came up to me and said, **"I know you're a Democrat, because Republican women don't have hair like yours."** I realized he was right, and I wonder which comes first: having curly hair and being a Democrat, or the other way around.

When I was young, people thought I was wild because of my hair. Curly hair definitely has that aura about it. I now live in New York, where there's more ethnic diversity, and different kinds of hair are more accepted. I'm a graphic artist and exhibition designer, and I don't think my hair is a professional liability. In fact, it's probably an asset, because it's so memorable. But I'm still pondering the question of which came first, the hair or the political affiliation.

—KATHLEEN TOBIN-JONES, GRAPHIC DESIGNER

LORRAINE'S LOTIONS AND POTIONS

If you hate putting all those chemicals from commercial products on your hair, try these homemade conditioners, rinses, and exfoliants that I've developed in my kitchen. You'll know they're fresh and natural because you make them yourself.

Lavender Mist

Lavender has cleansing properties, so this quick mist not only makes your hair smell like a lavender field in Provence, it's also indispensable for cleansing and reviving your curls. Make it in large quantities; keep a large spray bottle in your shower and smaller travel-size bottles in your purse, desk, and car.

1/2 gallon water
5 drops pure (not synthetic) lavender essential oil
3 empty spray bottles (available at most drugstores)

1. Fill a large pot with a half gallon of water.
2. Cover, bring to a boil, and simmer for an hour to get rid of impurities. (Check occasionally to make sure water isn't boiling away.)
3. Remove from heat, add lavender oil, stir, and replace lid.
4. Let steep until cool, then pour into empty spritz bottles.

Lavender mist makes a wonderful gift for friends, whether or not they are curly girls. Once you get hooked on the spray, you'll find lots of other uses for it. Some of my clients have told me that their husbands sprayed it on them in the delivery room, for a very calming effect.

Aloe Aroma Scalp Therapy

Aloe vera is a completely natural hydrating and conditioning therapy for your skin and scalp. The scalp is most responsive to this nourishing, cleansing treatment after it's been bathed in warm water and the pores are dilated.

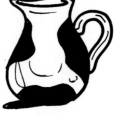

After you've rinsed or shampooed your hair in warm water, apply 1 tablespoon aloe vera gel to your scalp. (Use the edible type of aloe vera gel, the kind that has to be refrigerated after opening.) Massage gently for several minutes. Rinse hair and condition as usual. Or leave in, as an alternative to hair gel.

Deep-Pack Chakra

A calming protein pack to soften your hair, create bounteous curls, and nourish your spirit.

1 tablespoon powdered egg (found in health food stores)
1 tablespoon powdered milk
1/2 teaspoon honey (combined with a few drops of hot water to soften)
1–2 cups pasta water (for added nutrients) or plain boiled water
3 tablespoons heavy cream (optional)

1. Combine the first three ingredients to form a paste.

2. Add water (amount depends on the length and thickness of your hair).

3. Stir in fresh cream.

4. Pour the entire mixture over well-rinsed (but not freshly shampooed) hair.

5. Make a turban out of clear plastic wrap, wrap hair, and allow the rinse to penetrate for 1 hour or more, if possible.

6. Rinse well and condition, or shampoo and condition, depending on your hair type.

Lemon Aid

More clarifying and cleansing than any shampoo, this moisturizing and neutralizing tonic adds shine to your hair and removes buildup. It's especially good for very dry or damaged hair.

Combine juice of 1 large lemon with your usual amount of conditioner, then rinse through hair thoroughly.

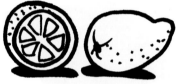

Deep Endings

A revitalizing oil treatment that nourishes the ends of your hair. It's especially useful in winter, when hair constantly rubs up against wool and other heavy fabrics.

> *1–3 teaspoons olive, peanut, or sweet almond oil (amount depends on length and/or thickness of your hair)*
> *2–4 drops pure lavender essential oil*

1. Combine oils and apply to the ends of your hair.

2. Wrap hair with clear plastic wrap and leave on for 30 minutes.

3. Rinse thoroughly with the Lemon Aid (above).

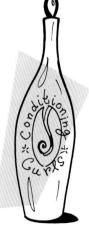

Most oil recipes tell you to shampoo afterward, but I think shampooing undermines the benefits of this treatment.

Avocado Wrap

Another rich moisturizing hair treat to nourish dry ends.

1 ripe avocado
3–4 teaspoons honey
8–10 drops almond oil

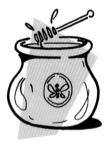

1. Peel and core the avocado, then mix in a blender with other ingredients.

2. Apply to wet hair, concentrating on the ends.

3. Wrap hair with clear plastic wrap or a towel. Leave on for 20–30 minutes.

4. Rinse thoroughly with warm water.

Whattacurl Wants

The baking soda will remove heavy product buildup and leave your hair feeling shiny and clean.

1 tablespoon baking soda
1 cup warm water

1. Combine above ingredients in a spray bottle and shake.

2. Wet, condition, and blot-dry hair as usual.

3. Spray with mixture.

4. Allow to sit for a minute or so, then rinse with cool water.

5. Blot dry again, style as usual.

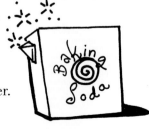

Flaking It

Excellent exfoliant for dry, flaking scalp.

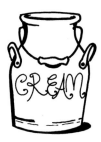

1 cup heavy cream, beaten until fluffy (or Reddi Whip)

Pour into palms and then massage into scalp. Wait 5–10 minutes, then rinse well with cool water.

Fruit Smoothie

A moisturizing and tasty banana cocktail that adds shine and bounce to dry or unruly curls.

3 very ripe bananas
1 teaspoon almond oil
½ cup carrot juice

1. Mix all three ingredients in a blender.

2. Apply to wet hair, making sure that all strands are well coated.

3. Wrap a damp towel around your head and leave on for a half hour.

4. Rinse thoroughly with warm (not hot) water.

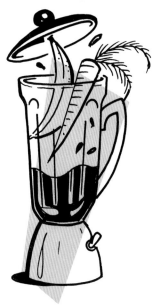

Love Is in the Hair

This sensual double dose of moisturizing oils acts as a refreshing tonic for dry, thirsty curls.

4 tablespoons olive or almond oil
4 tablespoons of your favorite conditioner
2–3 drops musk oil or other essential oil of your
    choosing

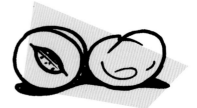

Mix well and apply to wet hair, combing through gently until your whole head is saturated. Use the entire amount for long hair, half the amount for short hair. Scrunch dry, then use clips to lift and separate the curls, as you would when styling. Leave in overnight or for several hours during the day. Rinse thoroughly with a combination of conditioner mixed with lemon juice and vinegar.

Curls from Ipanema

I was given this recipe by Ivone Da Silva, who has had over thirty years of experience as a hairstylist in Brazil. The potato starch–peach combination strengthens and revitalizes damaged, dry, or dull hair.

3 or 4 medium-size potatoes
2 cups water
1 peach (peeled)

1. Peel and wash potatoes, then cut them into chunks. Add water and refrigerate overnight in a covered bowl.

2. The next day, drain the water and save. (Discard the potatoes or add salt and pepper and cook for dinner.)

3. Puree the peach, then mix well with the potato water.

4. Apply the mixture to your hair and comb it through. Leave on for 20–30 minutes.

5. Rinse with water, and style as usual.

Glisten to Me

A gentle, all-natural hair spray that gives curls extra dimension and shine.

Vegetable glycerine (found at health food stores)
Distilled water (contains no minerals)
1 empty spray bottle (available at most drugstores)

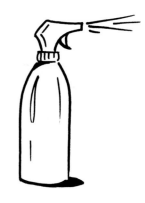

Combine equal parts of glycerine and water in a spritz bottle and mix. Spray whenever your hair looks dull or needs a quick pick-me-up.

Hair Dressing

Here's a fabulous trick that adds shine to your hair and eliminates frizz; it works best for Corkscrew and very dry Botticelli curls. Pick up one of those sleek-looking oil spray misters at your houseware specialty store. Fill it with olive oil and a few drops of your favorite perfume essence, then spray hair after it's dry. I love the effect so much that I now use the spray mister every few days, or whenever my hair looks or feels especially dry. For best results, use olive, canola, or any kind of nut oil.

When I was living in Israel over twenty years ago, my greatest wish—shared by my first husband—was that I have long, straight hair. Once a week, I would wash my natural curls and commit an entire evening to a straightening process, then popular among Israeli women, called *abuagela*.

Using large clips to hold it in place, I would painstakingly wrap my hair around one side of my head and sit under a hooded hair dryer for forty-five minutes. Then, just as painstakingly, I'd repeat the process on the other side of my head. During Israel's five-month rainy season, all I had to do was step outside, and the results would be totally undone. When I married my first husband, I had the *abuagela* done by a professional. With the torrential rains that day, I was terrified that my hair would get frizzy and ruin the wedding. The wedding photos attest to the power of the *abuagela*—my hair remained straight, at least through the ceremony.

First wedding: hair subjected to the abuagela.

I freed myself from this wrapping-and-drying bondage one very hot summer when I was living on a kibbutz near the Lebanese border. I went to a beauty parlor where Moroccan and Yemenite immigrants —women with hair far kinkier than my own—had their soft, beautiful curls cut very short. I returned to the kibbutz a changed woman, much to my husband's disapproval. That may have been the moment our marriage started to fall apart.

At my second wedding, which also took place in Jerusalem, **I wore my hair curly.** Fifteen years later, I'm still married to the same man and wear my hair wild and free, all different lengths and shades of blond. The spiraling curls spring in every direction, uninhibited by the dictates of any artificially imposed style—a perfect metaphor for how I now try to live my life.

—NAOMI CHIEL-BOLZMAN, EDUCATOR AND CANTORIAL STUDENT

Chapter Six

YOU GO, CURL!

African American Hair

"Eventually I knew what hair wanted;
it wanted to be itself . . . to be left alone
by anyone, including me, who
did not love it as it was."

—ALICE WALKER

Many of my curly girl clients are African American, and I tell them to follow my routine for caring for Corkscrew curls. They report particularly great results when they break the shampoo habit, which can cause serious damage to already dry hair and scalp that is a problem for the majority of African American women.

But I've also learned a great deal about curly hair care from them. For this chapter I've consulted with experts on African American hair and have asked a number of black women to tell their own hairstories. African American women have a lot to teach their curly-haired white sisters about hair care, including how often to wash it; how to hydrate very dry hair with conditioners and deep oil treatments; and what products to use.

Texturize and Hydrate

Joseph Plaskett Jr. is the co-owner of Joseph's, a family-run salon in Manhattan since 1958. Ninety percent of his clients are African American, but the shop often sees curly-haired white women, especially if they can't find a stylist who knows how to treat their corkscrew hair.

"If you want low-maintenance hair, natural is a good way to go," says Joseph. "If your hair is kinky, but you want a natural look, then you can soften and loosen the curl by texturizing it. We do a lot of texturizing in the salon, and the treatment does not damage the hair. I like an unstructured look, so if you have a good cut, you can just put some product in and rub your fingers through your hair—and let it do its thing.

"To keep hair healthy and shining, you need to hydrate the hair regularly with deep oil treatments, which most black women know because they grow up using pomades and oil treatments. At least once a week, apply vitamin E oil or an oil treatment to your scalp. (Any company that gears products to African Americans is going to have oil treatments.) Massage in, then comb through hair, using a wide-toothed comb. Preheat a heating cap and leave on for twenty minutes. Heat gives better penetration of the scalp. Then rinse thoroughly.

"In the salon, we like to do healthy things for African American hair," Joseph concludes. For example, instead of blow-drying hair or using curling irons, stylists roller-set the hair and put the client under the hair dryer. That way

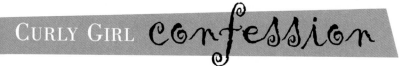

Growing up, I was ashamed of having nappy hair. Both my grandmother and my mother always wore straight wigs, and I learned early in life that my looks were not acceptable. When I was a youngster, in the fifties, my mother used to sit me down in the kitchen every Saturday night and hold a hot comb to my head—we called this "getting our hair pressed"— so I'd look presentable for church. I don't have any childhood pictures with my hair in its natural state, only straightened.

In the sixties, I grew the biggest Afro I could, modeling myself after Angela Davis, whom I worshiped. I'd argue with people who called the Afro a "hairstyle." "This isn't a style, it's a way of life!" I'd say. Later on, I grew my hair into locks, which I call Nubian. I wore them for about seven years, until they were almost to my waist.

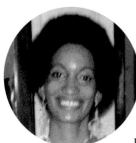

My Afro wasn't a "style"—it was a way of life.

I'd been thinking about cutting off the locks for about six months. **First, though, I talked to my hair, because I believe that hair has living energy.**

I said, "You're very pretty, and I really appreciate all you've done for me; it was fun to see how long you could grow. Now I have to let you go."

I now wear my hair cropped so close that you can see my scalp. When the hair starts to curl, I cut it off. (Actually, my husband cuts it with a pair of clippers we bought especially for this purpose.) I often ask myself, Why am I so intent on getting rid of the curls? Easy maintenance is part of it, but, also, I'm still caught up in ideas from my childhood of what hair is "supposed" to look like.

I used to obsess over having straight hair. I'm turning sixty this year, and now I'm working on not feeling that I have to look like someone else. **It's about attitude: if you're ashamed of your hair, you're not going to feel or look beautiful.** And as I start to appreciate myself as a person, I no longer see my hair as the summation of who I am. Like me, my hair is a work in progress.

—BARBARA WALTERS, CLINICAL SOCIAL WORKER

you use less heat to style hair, as opposed to the huge amount you use blow-drying hair from wet to dry.

Khamit Kurls Care

Annu Prestonia, owner of the Khamit Kurls salon in New York City, has specialized in African American hair care for over two decades. "Unlike curly hair, kinky hair that's more than an inch long must be combed or brushed before it's allowed to dry," says Annu. Otherwise "the hair gets tangled up in knots and mats together." She recommends using a rubber vent brush or comb to get rid of tangled hair, but only after the hair has been thoroughly wet and conditioned. Brush the hair out in small sections, twist or braid each section, then allow it to dry.

"We are a subtropical people," says Annu. "Where there's sun and warmth, we don't have problems with our scalp and skin. But cold-weather climates (and indoor heating) encourage dry scalp." She suggests moisturizing the hair and scalp two or three times a week, with conditioners formulated from natural plant- and herb-based ingredients, such as honeysuckle, oranges, and rosemary, as well as shea butter and coconut, jojoba, and olive oils. Just as I tell my clients, Annu recommends using lots of conditioner after washing your hair—much more than what's suggested on the bottle. If you have the time, wrap your head in plastic wrap and leave the conditioner on for an additional twenty minutes. Then rinse thoroughly, because conditioner tends to leave a visible film on kinky hair. Annu also recommends that clients dry their hair naturally, if at all possible.

Eighty percent of clients at Khamit Kurls come in for hair extensions, which can be worn braided, twisted, or loose. Why do so many African American

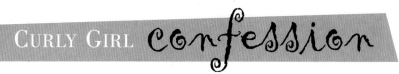
I never had what was considered "good" hair among African Americans, because mine was kinky rather than curly. I'd go to my aunt's beauty salon, where we'd have our hair "fried, dyed, and laid to the side."

Then came the era of the gigantic Afro. My mother was horrified when I had my hair cut in a 'fro. Women of her generation had fought, at great personal cost, to look white, respectable, middle class. And there I was, flaunting my kinky hair, looking like a hippie—or, worse, a revolutionary.

By the late eighties, Afrocentric hair was more acceptable. Women's magazines featured articles on curly hair, and there was an influx of immigrants from the Caribbean and East Africa. Among them were professional hairdressers who showed us how to achieve a sense of personal style.

When I remember what a degrading and humiliating process getting my hair straightened was, I wish I'd had a hair support group. For the last five years, I've worn my hair in extensions. They're worth the investment of time and money because they're so much easier to care for. I feel much freer now that I wear my hair in braids. They have a lot of movement and a wonderful sculptural shape that complements my wardrobe and makes me feel confident about my appearance.

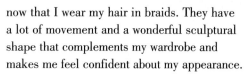

—JANICE BURGESS, TELEVISION PRODUCER

women opt for extensions, which can be a time-consuming and expensive process? I ask. "Our hair is strong but fragile," explains Annu. "Daily grooming eventually wears away at its vitality. Our ancestors, in their genius, came up with styles that allowed the hair to rest for periods of time and still look beautiful. As far back as ancient Egypt, African women and men had extensions."

Today, African American women are just as likely to choose braids or locks because they want to preserve the health of their hair. And braids are a style whose time has definitely come.

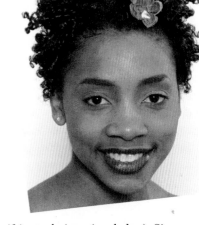

When I do stage work I usually wear a wig, but when I go on auditions, I wear my hair natural. Most of the black women you see in commercials these days have curly hair—it's very "in" now.

I'm from a Jamaican background, where natural hair comes with a lot of stigma, but I'm not trying to make a political statement with my hair. (Though people often want me to.) A lot of black women get perms because they think it makes their hair more manageable.

A few years ago, when I had a perm, my hair was very thin and damaged and my scalp was very dry. My hair wasn't healthy, so **I started growing it out and wore extensions through the transitional period.** After I had two or three inches of natural hair, I took out the extensions and cut off the permed ends.

If I wash my hair and go, it tends to get really matted and I'm not able to put a comb through it when it's dry. I set my hair in straws as an antifrizz technique (see below). Since I've gone natural, my hair is much stronger. I wear my hair curly because I like the way it looks.

—SIMONE MOORE, ACTRESS AND MODEL

Simone's Straw Set

Simone Moore shared this straw set styling technique, which she uses to prevent frizz. It works best for short hair. (Hers is only three inches long all over.) You'll need: styling gel, plastic drinking straws (she cuts them in half; but if your hair is longer, you may want to use whole straws), and bobby pins.

After wetting and conditioning hair, comb it out using a wide-toothed comb, then apply styling gel to hair.

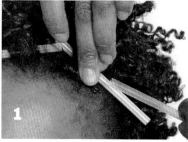

1. Holding the straw as you would a ruler, take a one-inch section of hair and gently roll the strand onto the straw, up and away from your forehead. Make sure you position the straw vertically, or at right angles to your scalp.

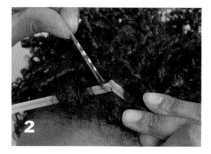

2. Insert a bobby pin through one end of the straw to secure.

3. Set hair in rows, working from the front of your head to the back. When you finish setting all of your hair, the straws will be in a pinwheel pattern. Allow your hair to air-dry or sit under a dryer for thirty minutes.

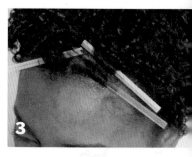

4. When you first take the straws out, the result may be too much of a Shirley Temple look for you, but then you can fingerstyle to loosen the curls. When dry, your hair is shiny and curly, rather than kinky.

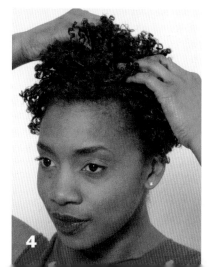

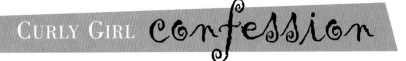
My hair falls somewhere between kinky frizz and perfect curls. My sister, who has big, silky ringlets that I have always coveted, took charge of our hair when she was seven and I was five because my mother, whose hair is blond and straight, had no experience dealing with "mixed girl's hair."

My sister was very particular about doing our hair correctly. That meant putting it in two tight braids, the way all the other little girls—the black girls—put their hair up, and still do. But you didn't *just* put it in two braids; it was a real process. First, she'd part my hair perfectly—and I mean perfectly—down the middle. Then she'd use a brush specifically for coarse hair that made my scalp hurt. She'd use the elastic bands with the two colorful plastic balls attached and tie them extremely tight around the ends of both braids.

For a while we had a black nanny living with us. She was the epitome of everything I'd felt I was missing. Because I never had a black mom, I'd look to her for how to do my hair. We'd go to church with her, and she'd pull my hair back so hard that my eyelids would stretch and I felt as if my eyeballs would pop out.

At nine, I decided that I wanted to choose my own hairstyle, and

My sister took charge of our hair when I was five.

my mom brought me to a white-girl salon to get my hair relaxed. It was a big ordeal: they didn't know quite what to do with me. Once I started going to black hair salons the process turned out a little better—much straighter than the first time. I wore my hair straight, getting it done every two weeks, until my sophomore year of high school, when I attempted to wear it curly. When I got to school that day, one of my black friends told me that it looked like a dry Jheri-curl. Some white classmates said, "Your hair looks so cool." They thought that I had gotten a perm.

I really believe that when you wear your hair curly, everything starts falling into place. It's easier and natural. Today both African American and white people tell me they love my hair. **I'm lucky, because this is a good time to have curly hair.** It's considered cool now, and at twenty-two, I finally know how to take care of it.

—**HILARY MITCHELL, TELEVISION PRODUCTION ASSISTANT**

Chapter Seven

A CUTTING-EDGE PHILOSOPHY

A Crop of Curls

A stylist must approach each head and each curl as a separate entity with a mind of its own.

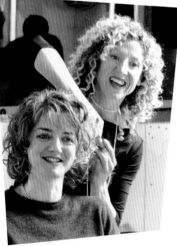

Getting a haircut is one of life's most traumatic moments for curly girls. No matter where you live, you've had at least one bad haircut in your life, maybe a lot more than that. You've asked for a trim and ended up completely shorn and looking like a skinned poodle; you've had an inexperienced stylist wet your hair down, then cut it as though it's straight, and you've ended up with mismatched and unflattering layers of angry curls. I've gone home in tears after a haircut, and so has almost every other curly girl in the world. So when a nervous customer sits down in front of me for the first time, I tell her I know where she's coming from. I explain her history so thoroughly, she thinks I've been spying on her. (Whatever our background, all curly girls share a common language about our hair.)

I begin by telling her that I'm going to give her a haircut that's just for her. Everyone's curly hair is different—in the tightness of curls, in how randomly the curls are distributed, and in how they grow naturally and frame the face. You'll never find the right cut in one of those books of styles that some salons pass around as if you're ordering a meal. You can't do that with curly hair.

In other words, there is no "style" for curly heads. I can't hand you a picture and say that's how you're going to look. You've been blessed with hair that has a mind of its own. Every strand is a separate entity that reacts differently to the scissors. The stylist has to approach each curl individually, considering its texture, its degree of curliness, and how it relates to the curls around it. I don't wet hair before a cut because I know that's a sure way to cut too much. Lopping off two inches all around on a curly head can leave the hair *five or six* inches shorter when the hair is dry. Cutting curly hair is about what you leave, not what you snip off.

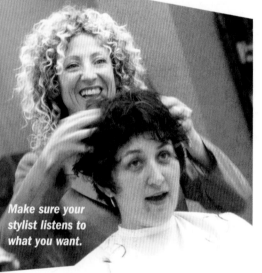

Make sure your stylist listens to what you want.

I recently led a hair workshop for professional stylists on new and advanced styling and coloring techniques. Of the fifty or so men and women in the room, at least twenty-five had curly hair. I asked the curly heads how many of them had blow-dried their hair that day. At least ten people raised their hands. When I asked why, almost everyone said that blowing their hair straight was easier than trying to deal with curls. Finally, I asked how many of them *liked* their curls.

One woman stood up and said she could learn to love her curly hair if she could get it to look like mine. Most of the others nodded in agreement.

I wasn't surprised by their responses. I've yet to attend a hairdressing workshop in the United States that offered instructions on understanding and cutting curly hair, and I've seen very few curly-haired models participating in hairdressing seminars or classes.

In England, where the instruction is more comprehensive than what's offered in the United States, the emphasis is on cause and effect, explaining why certain techniques are preferable to others, and how every head

What lies beneath the canopy is a clue to what kind of cut a curly girl needs.

of hair requires an individualized approach. Each client has a different degree of movement and texture, a different hairline, a different cowlick. Curly hair is not predictable, which makes it impossible to categorize types of cuts. English and European stylists tend to cut hair dry, which makes excellent sense, for the simple reason that that's how we wear our hair. *It's also the only way to cut curly hair.*

My first-time clients are surprised when I don't send them off to have their hair washed immediately. Instead, I begin by asking the client to sit up straight in the chair, so I can examine her hair carefully. I pay attention to every movement, every contour, every characteristic. Is the hair frizzy? Overly dry? Stiff or crispy from too much gel or other products? Has it been straightened and dried out by blow-drying? Is the curl on the left side of the face tighter than the curl on the right side? Are the bangs begging for a trim? I listen to the client, but I also allow her hair to "tell" me its story, to let me know what its needs are.

I trim the curl a little at the ends to reduce frizz.

I next moisten the hair with lavender spray and scrunch it gently so that I can figure out the client's type of curl. Sometimes, especially if the hair has been blown dry, it needs a thorough wetting, so I have the client's hair washed with conditioner, scrunched, and dried under a heat lamp. Only then do I begin the actual cutting process.

Unless the client wants a much shorter look, which happens very rarely, most curly haircuts are about maintenance after the initial cut. Curls need to "read" their natural length. When I'm working on Corkscrew or Botticelli curls, I unfurl each curl and examine it as a separate entity, looking for frayed ends. I decide on the minimum amount that needs to be trimmed, then cut at the beginning of each curl to maintain its shape and avoid any

Magic Touch

An appointment with Lorraine is much more than a haircut. We talk about self-exploration and life issues, not just celebrity gossip. There's almost something magical about the way she touches my hair; I think it's because she really respects it.

—NATHALIE WECHSLER, CLIENT

Cut the curl at the beginning of each C.

dramatic spring-back. Think of a natural curl as an *S* shape. *S*'s are *C*'s reversed and sitting on top of each other. I cut the curl at the beginning of each *C*. While I'm cutting, I constantly shake the curls from the root to see where they lie and how they're going to fall when they're in motion, something you can't do when they're wet. And I try never to cut too much.

What's your natural length? It's that point when your curls flatter your face and fall gracefully. Some people need to grow their curls to shoulder length before the natural pattern of their curls emerges. Others have curls that can be cut shorter. I ask the client what length she's happiest with and try to accommodate her preference. In general, it's better for the client to leave the salon upset because her hair is too long rather than too short.

I start by pulling down the hair on either side of the face to make sure that it's even. I then look for pairs of curls or waves, which I call "Siamese twins"— a thick, heavy top layer of curls that is drooping and weighing down the curls beneath it. I divide a thick curl into two layers and trim one slightly shorter. The pattern and length of the exterior curl or wave is maintained, but it becomes bouncier because its load has been lightened. The newly shortened layer of curl pushes the longer curl outward and keeps it buoyant. In other words, the shorter curls support the longer curls and add volume to the hair.

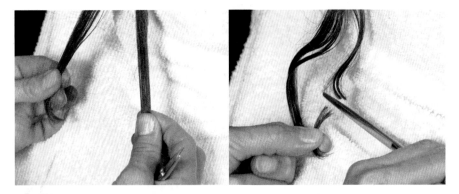

To add volume: I divide a thick curl into two and trim one shorter.

This "super-in-position" method can also be used for curls that are top-heavy (i.e., all growing out at the same time).

You don't want bilevel curls, where the top layer looks as if it doesn't belong to the bottom layer. If the top layer of curls is still short, let it grow awhile. What you do want are seamless layers, which begin no higher than your chin. Tight curly hair tends to balloon out in an east-west direction, so that all the width of the hairdo is someplace around your chin. A cutter has to shape the curls carefully so this doesn't happen.

Above all, don't despair. If you find a stylist (see "Finding the Kindest Cut—and Cutter," pages 75–78) who's willing to listen to your hair needs and cut your hair dry, you will see a change. If a stylist has taken off too much, it may take six months before you really like your hair again. Be patient, follow my routine for conditioning and cleansing your hair—and your curls will heal themselves.

Finding the Kindest Cut
—and Cutter

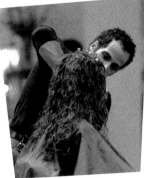

You've come this far. You're a certified curly girl and you know how to care for your hair. It looks and feels better than it ever has. Now you have to find a good stylist, someone who can trim and shape your curls. Get the wrong person and all your hard work will be literally swept off the cutting room floor. Here are some of the things to think about and ask before you let anyone approach your hair with a scissors.

As every curly girl knows, finding a stylist who understands your hair is harder than finding a brain surgeon or a good defense attorney. The surest way, of course, is to see a haircutter's work. So when you spot someone with curly hair that looks wonderful, ask her where she has it cut. (Don't hesitate because you think it's intrusive; most people will be flattered by the question.) If you live in New York or Los Angeles, you might flip through

Curly Cut Dos and Don'ts

- ☐ *DO cut the hair when it is dry.*
- ☐ *DO avoid blunt cuts, which ignore the spring factor and stretch the hair to an unnatural state so it's too short when it dries.*
- ☐ *DO cut just before the crest of each curl.*
- ☐ *DO the top front of the hair last, and DON'T take too much off here because the curls are shortest and most fragile there.*
- ☐ *DON'T overly layer the hair.*
- ☐ *DON'T thin out fine curly hair. The gravity/weight of a strong curl is what gives hair definition.*
- ☐ *DON'T use a razor to cut curly hair. It isn't as sharp as scissors and can create badly frayed ends.*

magazines for a style you like, then check the credits for the name of the salon or stylist. Otherwise, keep asking around until you find someone whose hair looks great. Next step, phone the salon and ask the following questions:

- ☐ Is the stylist an expert at cutting curly hair?

- ☐ Does the stylist have naturally curly hair? Does she wear it curly? If so, this is a good sign.

- ☐ Will the stylist see you for a consultation? Don't be offended if the answer is no—it could mean she's so popular that she has no time. Some places charge for a consultation.

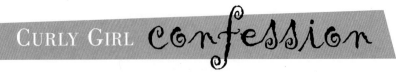

CURLY GIRL *confession*

For the last fifteen years or so, I wore my hair in long ringlets that cascaded down my back. **I cut my hair short twice—both times because I was involved with men who loved my hair long and they pissed me off. Men put so much value on hair.**

A couple of years ago, I was thinking about cutting my hair because my face had gotten thinner, I'd lost my chubby cheeks, and the long hair look wasn't doing it for me anymore. I'd been in a relationship for six years with a much younger boyfriend, a Frenchman, and we'd been trying to break it off for forever. When he went back to France, I did it. I had my ringlets cut off. The new, much shorter length felt cathartic and liberating.

Then my boyfriend called to say he wanted me to come to Paris for a visit. "You wouldn't want to see me," I told him. "I had all my hair chopped off." There was complete silence on the other end of the telephone. Finally he got up the nerve to ask why. "Because I can," I said.

—LEONTINA LANGE, CLOTHING DESIGNER

☐ Does the salon offer the option of drying the hair under heat lamps rather than with blow-dryers? Explain that you want to keep your hair curly.

☐ Does the stylist cut very curly hair while it's dry? If the answer is no, is he willing to listen and be open to a different approach? Unless a stylist can see how much spring there is in your curls, he won't understand your hair and he's likely to cut too much when it's wet, only to discover that fact after your hair dries.

☐ What products does the salon use? If you don't use shampoo and have a favorite conditioner, bring it with you and, politely, say that you prefer them to use it. Most stylists won't object, especially if your hair is in good condition.

Let's assume you got all the right answers and have made an appointment. But if, when you arrive, you're told to change and get your hair shampooed, a "bad hair" alert bell should go off. Instead, the stylist should sit you down, examine your hair, touch it, talk with you about your hair and what you envision having done—all before picking up the scissors. Pull a typical curl down to its farthest point and let go, so the stylist can see how tight the curl is. If your curls vary in tightness, show her which ones have a smaller spring factor. This is important so that she doesn't cut too much. Finally, explain that you'd rather leave your hair a bit too long than go too short.

Ideally, after the cut, the stylist should wet your hair and let it dry to see the finished results. This is the point when he or she makes those all-important final touches, picking up split ends that were missed the first time around or adjusting how the curls fall. You may want him to handpick and cut a few curls, especially around the front of your face.

Don't be afraid to talk to the stylist about your preferences, as long as you're polite. If this is a friendly neighborhood place, he may be happy to work with you and talk about curly hair problems. If this is a trendy big-city salon, your stylist may have an attitude problem, so be diplomatic but firm. After all, whose hair is it, anyway?

CURLY GIRL *confession*

People treat you more seriously when you have straight hair. They think curly hair is unprofessional. They want you to look tame and corporate, like an anchor-woman, with "anchor hair."

My five-year-old daughter, Josie, also has curly hair, but it's finer than mine and not as curly. She is thrilled when it's straight because most of her friends have straight hair. She also wants bangs, but if I let her have them, they'd curl up toward her fore-head and look goofy, sort of like Hayley Mills in *The Parent Trap.*

I wear my hair curly when I'm rebellious and want to make a statement. It's my free-spirited, hippie look. It means I'm my own person, a solo flyer, and I don't have to conform to anyone's view of what a mother and working professional should look like.

—LUCY DANZIGER, MAGAZINE EDITOR

Chapter Eight

COLOR ME CURLY

The Best Choices for Curls

By now, you're an expert on curly hair. You know how it differs from straight hair, you know that it requires special cutting and care, and you've learned how to live with it. Now that your daily routine nurtures your hair, you might want to shake things up a bit and experiment with your look by adding highlights or color.

Yes, color and curls *do* mix, especially now with the range of available color processes that can keep hair healthy looking. But you must take into account the special needs of curly hair and use color gently and sensibly. Curly hair absorbs damaging chemicals more easily because the cuticle around the hair shaft is open. "It also takes longer to recover from any damage, because the hair is so porous," says Denis DaSilva, the co-owner of Devachan. He and Shari Harbinger are the salon's color experts, and I consider them among the best colorists in the country.

Denis and Shari recommend using either semipermanent or demipermanent colors as the best choices for curly hair. "Semipermanent is not as damaging to the hair because it doesn't remove any of the natural color," says Shari. And the fewer ammonia-based products we use on our hair, the less dehydrated it becomes. Demipermanent color, however, is more effective on gray hair that may resist a milder coloring process.

At Devachan, we usually recommend that clients come back every four to six weeks for semipermanent color. Six weeks after the initial color treatment, we need to refresh the roots as well as the ends of the hair shaft. Beyond that period, most of the color will have faded or washed out.

Curly girls, especially those who have Corkscrew curls, should avoid dramatic color transformations overnight. Start with a demi- or semipermanent color that's close to your own, or two or three tones lighter. Live with it for a while before doing anything more drastic. Remember that all hair, but particularly curly hair, takes at least a week to recover from the trauma of being treated, and the depth and dimension of color will change as the curls return to their normal state.

As I often tell my clients, blond shouldn't be built in a day. If you do want to go from dark brown to blond, you need to build in the color over time. A couple of years ago, I decided I wanted a dramatic change. I waited until I knew for sure that my curls—and I—could deal with it, then chose a "good curl day"—a day when my hair looked great and I was feeling upbeat. I opted for a less caustic lightener and began by having just a few handpicked curls highlighted. I loved the results and the positive feedback I was getting, so I went for a full-blown lightening treatment. Now, I'm ready for a slightly different image; I'm going to introduce more "low lights," darker strands throughout the hair that will create contrasting colors. The result should be even more dramatic.

Even with semipermanent colors, the hair may lose some shine after coloring. Sometimes, after a color treatment, we use a gloss, a silicone-based product that restores shine and adds polish to the surface of the hair. We recommend glosses with a hint of color because they're more reflective and make hair richer and healthier looking. Glosses are a good choice, too, for gray hair that needs to look a little less yellow and more vibrant. They'll seal the cuticle, blend your gray hair, or make it shine like well-polished silver.

If you're in the mood for drama, you can have fun playing with highlights a few shades brighter than your natural color. At Devachan, we specialize in *pintura*, a highlighting technique invented by Denis. "The best way to highlight curly hair is to paint it on while the hair is dry," he says. "Painting is so visual that you need to see what you're doing to the hair."

"You're creating light on a canvas where there is no light," says Shari, "and you're defining the design of the cut." Curly hair is best for painting, because the colorist can pick out the more raised pieces of

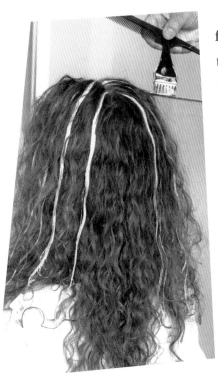

Pintura *coloring will give definition to your curls.*

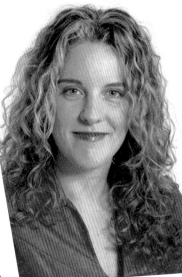

hair—the ones that best reflect the light. So you're guaranteed that you'll see the highlights exactly where you paint them. "If you paint the highlighted pieces too closely together," continues Shari, "you lose dimension, which curly hair needs. I leave a lot of space between each ribbon of light that

After: *subtly brighter*

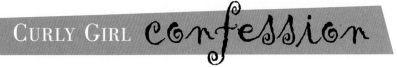
When I was growing up, I was obsessed with the story of Rapunzel and her long hair. I loved giving my long-haired dolls different hairstyles, because my parents forced me to keep my own hair short. They thought curls were meant to be tamed. **There is something about lots of curly hair that's very sexual, and parents don't like to see that in their kids.** My parents wanted me to behave like a nice, quiet girl from a good family. So I kept my hair "quiet," but I rebelled in *other* ways.

Then as soon as I was out on my own, I let my hair grow out and go wild. I now think that **my fascination with Rapunzel's hair has to do with becoming powerful and feeling in control.** Rapunzel's long hair gave her the power to escape from the tower. I grew my hair long when my parents were no longer able to control me—or my curls.

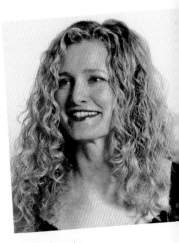

Today I work at an Internet company, where everyone else has tattoos and pierced body parts, so my wild hair is totally okay. In fact, people expect me to look unusual. People are fascinated by my curls; strangers stop me on the street, and many even ask to touch it. However, some things never change: even though I'm now thirty-six, my parents are still trying to "fix" my appearance. I'll be talking to my father, and he'll say in that tone, "Get your hair out of your face."

—NATHALIE WECHSLER, INTERNET COMPANY EXECUTIVE

I paint, so when the hair curls and sits away from the head, you see the contrast between the lighter and darker strands."

Before you have your hair colored, treat it very gently for a few weeks. Keep up the daily conditioning, and if you still shampoo, don't do it near the day of your color treatment. The harsh detergents in shampoos exacerbate the damaging effects of coloring. If you're opting for a new style, or getting your hair trimmed and shaped, get your hair cut first, then colored. After you get color, treat your hair with special TLC, using one of the moisturizing treatments recommended in chapter 5 (see pages 53–59). Remember that the more often you shampoo your hair, the more quickly the color will fade. (Another good reason not to shampoo!) You may want to use a color conditioner or mousse to minimize fading. Ask your colorist what he or she recommends. We sometimes custom-mix conditioning products for our clients, and your salon may offer a similar service.

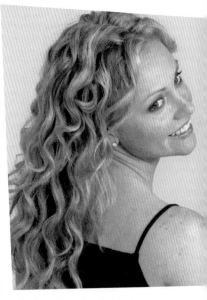

Curls painted individually resemble ribbons of light.

Clients often ask me what I think about do-it-yourself coloring. Shari, Denis, and I all give a thumbs-down to the idea of home coloring. "If you have a discerning eye and artistic hand, it could work," says Shari. "But it takes longer for curly hair to recover from lost moisture than straight hair, so why take the chance?"

Denis agrees. "For curly girls, coloring kits can be a nightmare. The hair companies may call their products semipermanent, but the ingredients in home kits are the chemical equivalent of almost permanent color. Your hair is already dry and tends to frizz, so don't put it at risk by using overly strong solutions. You may think you'll save money, but if your hair is long, you'll end up spending more money than you might expect."

CURLY GIRL *confession*

I grew up in a Turkish ghetto in Germany, one of eight children, and my mother used to give us all haircuts every six weeks. After I discovered that I had curls, I rebelled and started growing out my hair. By the time I was thirteen, it was thick and curly and reached to my hips. I have four very beautiful sisters, but I was the one with the beautiful hair.

My father used to taunt me, "If you didn't have your hair, you'd have to kill yourself, because you're ugly." His words hurt so much that one day when I was fourteen, I grabbed a pair of garden shears and chopped off all my hair, just to show him I didn't give a damn about beauty.

When I was in art school I went to my first hairdresser and had my hair dyed bright red, which was a real novelty in Germany in 1986. The other students, who loved to touch it, taunted me with the name *rote Hexe*—the red witch. But I liked that label.

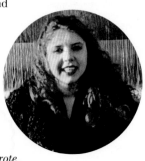

Women in the German-Turkish ghetto where I grew up must ask their husband's permission before they can cut their hair. I've noticed that the first thing Turkish women do when they come to America is chop off their hair and straighten it. **When I moved to New York City, everyone told me to tie my hair back to get jobs, especially in the corporate world.** I straightened my hair only twice, and both times I got treated with more respect, as if I were a lady. My curly hair makes me more approachable, and men think they can talk to me in a freer way.

My curls tell a lot about me. Some days, if I don't feel good about myself, my hair just hangs there, as droopy as my spirits. Other days, if I'm happy or in love, my hair bounces and looks shiny. I've been getting a lot of compliments lately about my hair—things must be looking up!

—GÜLER UĞUR,
PHOTOGRAPHER

Chapter Nine

THE CARE AND HANDLING OF CURLY KIDS

Getting Kids to Like Their Curls

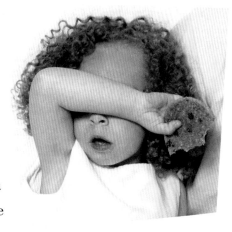

"Daddy says that Amy looks like a little Greek goddess with her thick, black curls," is the very first entry in Amy Helfman's baby journal. I don't know what the later entries are, but I can guess one: "Amy's mom says that Amy's curly hair is driving her crazy." If you're the parent of a curly-haired kid, as I am, or if you've been one yourself, you know what I'm talking about. Curly hair can get into more messes than a two-year-old with a bucket of chocolate.

Kids are constantly running, tumbling, swinging, and jumping into mud puddles and piles of leaves. They throw sand at one another. They plop winter hats, dress-up hats, and baseball caps on top of their heads and never worry about whether their curls get matted or snarled. Until it comes time to wash those curls. Then oceans of tears get washed down the drain along with the sand and dirt.

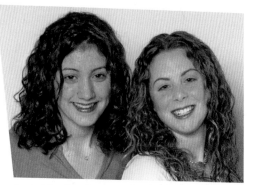

Best friends mirror each other; when Karly (right) stopped ironing her hair, so did Justine. Now they talk every day about their curls.

I recommend treating kids' curly hair the same way I treat adults' hair. My younger son has very curly hair, and I stopped using shampoo on his hair about the same time I stopped using it on my own. If I notice a dry patch on his scalp, I massage it gently with olive oil. He's never had cradle cap (a yellowish crust that often develops on infant scalps), and both his hair and his scalp look healthy and smell clean.

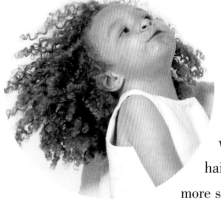

While baby shampoos usually are manufactured with detergents that are milder than most, it's still a good idea to *dilute the shampoo* with spring or distilled water before using it. Apply a small amount to the scalp and massage lightly. Resist the urge to work a generous amount of lather directly onto the hair, which will only ruffle the shaft and create even more snarls than already exist.

Ask your child to look up at the ceiling as you rinse the hair with water. Try to pour the water in the direction that the hair is growing, to help smooth the tangles and evenly distribute the shampoo. Continue rinsing until the water runs clear and you're satisfied that the shampoo has been flushed away.

Apply conditioner. If your child has baby-fine hair, use only a very small amount of conditioner, perhaps as little as a quarter teaspoon, or apply it only to the ends of the hair. Comb it through wet hair, beginning at the ends, and gently work your way up, using either a medium-toothed comb or your fingers to separate the tangles. (Never use a brush, which can turn the curls into a mass of frizz.) Rinse thoroughly, then reapply another quarter to half teaspoon of conditioner, depending on the texture and length of the curls.

Just Checking, Mom

My hair is like the waves, my hair is like the rug—curly zigzags. None of my friends has curly hair. My best friend has straight blond hair. I always ask my mom, "How do I get hair like that?"

My mom's the only one I know who's curlier than me. She says she loves her hair. Some days I ask her, "Do you still like your hair?—Just checking, Mom."

—**Izzy Mandel, age 7**

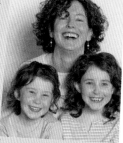

Izzy (right) with mom and sister, Sophie.

If your curly-haired daughter insists on wearing her hair straight, comb it and put it in a ponytail to dry. Or braid the hair while it's still wet, which will help eliminate frizz. For curly styles, blot dry with a towel, apply a small amount of gel, and scrunch, as described in "Curls on the Go," page 45.

You can make your own detangling spray by combining an equal amount of water and conditioner in a spray bottle. This works wonders on curly kids' hair, which is healthier and more hydrated than ours so their curls usually don't need full-strength conditioning. Use your judgment: older girls with long, thick curls will need more conditioner than a younger child with short, fine hair.

What happens when your curly kid comes home with glue, paste, or a wad of gum in her hair? Rub the area with an ice cube until the sticky mess hardens and begins to crumble, then dab on a few drops of vinegar and about half a teaspoon of condi-

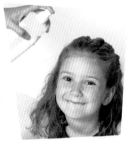

tioner, depending on the size of the substance. Gently work it out with your fingers, rinse with the detangling spray, and comb through again, using more conditioner, if necessary.

My kids are used to my spritzing them with Lavender Mist (see recipe on page 53). It's great in the morning when they wake up with ruffled hair. I also use it to give their hair a quick rinse after a day at the beach. A little-known side benefit for school-age kids: the lavender spray is a great deterrent against lice.

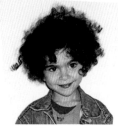

Cut #2: short bob with bangs

Cozy Wolan, owner of Cozy's Cuts for Kids in New York City, usually assigns curly-haired stylists the job of cutting curly kids' hair. She and I agree that kids need haircuts that simplify grooming. "Most kids won't sit still for more than two seconds when they're having their hair combed, so a child's haircut shouldn't require styling or blow-drying," she says.

I suggest two basic styles for curly kids. You can go for a very free and natural look, allowing the hair to follow its intrinsic shape, whether waves, ringlets, or smaller curls. This works very well for both girls and boys, although older boys are apt to resist a head of ringlets, no matter how charming it looks to you. For very easy care, cut your little curly girl's hair in a short bob with bangs. Keep the hair all one length, but allow a bit of an east-west direction—

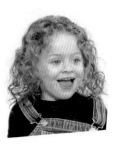

Cut #1: free and natural

it looks adorable on little girls.

Getting Kids to Like Their Curls

Luckily for curly kids today, curls are in! Magazines that once showed nothing but straight lank hair now do features on how you can make your straight hair curly—quite a fashion reversal! But old prejudices die hard, and some kids are still made to feel that their curls are different, weird, funny. Cozy has tiny clients who come in regularly to have their hair blown straight. "I don't know where it comes from," she says. "But I see kids of five or six who are unhappy about their curls."

My own clients frequently tell me that they hated their curls from a very young age. And only a few years ago, I met a little girl who couldn't have been more than four years old whose father told me, "She hates her curls, so we try to point out women who have beautiful curly hair." The child had a head of gorgeous ringlets, but when I complimented her on them, she frowned at me and hid her head in her father's coat. It can be a casual remark, made in the child's company, or just the fact of making too much of a small child's hair. But children are quick to pick up on prejudices of all kinds.

Take advantage of today's trend to point out the benefits of curls to your own curly tops. But don't make a big deal out of it, or they'll figure something's up. Instead, once in a while, point out a woman with beautiful curly hair. Or talk about how much you like your own curls.

If you have straight hair and your child is curly, find her a curly-haired mentor—someone she can bond with over hair, its glory, its problems, and its orneriness. I might have avoided years of agony, especially during my adolescence, if only I'd known a curly girl to talk to. I'd spend hours in front of the mirror sobbing because I looked so hideous. When it was really humid, I'd wear my brother's balaclava, a woolen cap that fit skintight.

That's why I try to be a mentor to any curly-haired child or teenager who needs it. I think my teenage years would have been very different if only an enlightened curly girl had taken me under her wing and said, "Call me if you have any questions about how to take care of your curls."

If You're Straight and Your Kid Is Curly . . .

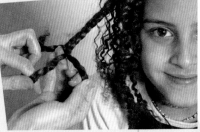

I'm white, and my husband is black. Our daughter, Naisha, has very thick, kinky hair. I didn't have a clue about how to treat her hair when she was a baby, so I left it short and curly until she was about a year and a half old. Then a friend said, **"You better learn how to take care of it, so people won't think you're a white mom who doesn't know how to deal with black hair."** About that time, a Caribbean woman started baby-sitting for Naisha, and she showed me how to create cornrows that kept her hair from getting matted. Generations of black women have taught one another how to care for their kinky hair. When you're grafted onto the culture, you have to find someone, as I did, to advise you.

Naisha is eight now, and my routine for maintaining her shoulder-length hair takes at least an hour and a half. After I shampoo and comb out her hair, using lots of conditioner, I set her up in front of a video and start sectioning the hair to make cornrows. It's a bit of an ordeal, especially as her hair begins to dry and gets tangled more easily. When we're finished, I often ask her, "Was it worth the pain? Would you want to do it again?" Up to now, her answer has been yes.

Although Naisha says she loves how her hair looks, she says if she had a magic wand, she'd give herself straight blond hair. That's so ironic, because as a little girl, I didn't like my hair because it was thin and stringy. I thought the black girls who wore the braided styles were really neat. Now I enjoy making cornrows, and I sometimes tell Naisha that taking care of her hair "is a privilege and a treat."

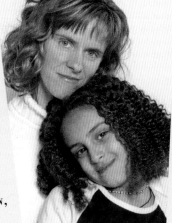

—PATRICIA HOGAN,
OCCUPATIONAL
THERAPIST

Chapter Ten

CURLY GIRL Q & A

No More Bad Hair Days

Q: What can I do for an itchy scalp?

A: This may sound flip, but my first answer is: Scratch it! An occasional itch is perfectly normal and doesn't necessarily signify a problem. Our skin constantly responds to stimuli in the environment. As I'm writing this sentence, the little finger of my left hand feels itchy, yet my skin looks perfectly healthy and rash-free.

If you're recovering from a longtime addiction to shampoo, your scalp will probably feel itchy a couple of days after you stop using it. An itch is often a sign that your scalp is healing, much like a scab does before it begins to heal. Though your scalp is starting to heal from a constant state of dehydration, an itch is a signal that it needs still more moisture.

If you have severely dry hair, make the Exfoliating Scrub on page 38. Wet your hair thoroughly, then massage in the scrub. If you tend to have combination skin and hair, wet the hair and give your scalp a massage without the conditioner. Start at the hairline using a circular motion. First, tackle the sides and crown and then move down to the nape of the neck. Repeat the treatment every three days for a week.

You can also try spot-cleaning (see page 33) or spritzing your scalp with Lavender Mist (see page 53), which contains natural medicinal properties that help cleanse the skin.

If the itching continues or becomes more severe, consult a dermatologist.

Q: My hair looks dull. How can I get it to shine?

A: First, how long have you been following my curly hair treatment routine? Give it two or three weeks before you expect miracles.

Your hair responds to the way you treat it. What are you doing to your hair that might cause dullness? Give up the myth that brushing one hundred strokes a night is good for your hair and donate your hairbrush to someone who needs it, maybe your cat or dog. Brushing can damage the cuticle of curly hair and rob it of its sheen.

If your hair really does appear dull, consider getting a semipermanent gloss for added shine. The gloss coats and seals the hair shaft so that it looks shinier than usual. You can get this treatment at a salon, and it will keep your hair shining for weeks. (See page 80.)

By the way, before deciding your hair is too dull, check out the light in your bathroom. We often judge ourselves based on what we see as we're standing in a small bathroom that's lit by fluorescent light directly above our heads. Try looking in a mirror when you're outside in natural light. This will give you a much better idea of the true state of your hair.

A: Hair grows half an inch a month, sometimes even as much as an inch a month. If you can't get to the salon when you need a touch-up, try camouflaging your roots by using the crossover trick:

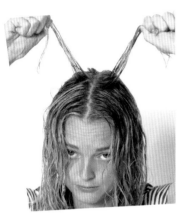

Part your hair, then pick out two small sections of hair at the middle of the crown, on either side of the part. Cross the strands over each other, and pin

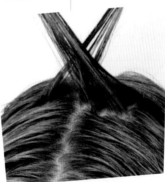

into place with a bobby pin. Continue working your way toward your forehead, until you've covered the part with three or four sections of hair. If you do this while your hair is wet, the sections will dry unevenly and cover up the part where the roots show. The idea is to create a landscape of mini hills and valleys that provides natural cover for your roots. In a pinch, you can use mascara on the roots. (They now make "hair mascara" in light and dark shades just for this purpose.)

Q: I'm pregnant. What changes can I expect in my hair?

A: I see many women whose hair is fuller and bouncier during pregnancy, but the front of their hair breaks more easily. You can restore the health of your hair after your baby is born by cutting off some of the length. About three to eight months after you give birth, or after you've stopped breast-feeding, your hair may show signs of breakage. Instead of your usual trim, cut off a couple of inches. This will decrease the weight pulling on the follicles.

If you notice that your hair won't grow past a certain point, it may have less to do with your pregnancy and more to do with your hair routine. Overwashing, brushing, or too much coloring can fray the ends and cause the hair to break.

Q: I swim in a pool three or four times a week. How is the chlorine affecting my curly hair?

A: You can judge how high a pool's chlorine levels are by how quickly the color of your bathing suit begins to fade. Imagine what that does to your hair. If you plan to spend the day at the pool, mix up a pint of distilled water with a table-spoon of conditioner and put it in a spray bottle. Spritz as soon as you get out of the pool.

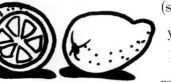

You absolutely do not have to shampoo your hair after swimming in a chlorinated pool, because that just subjects your hair to more drying chemicals and dehydration. Instead, flush thoroughly with water when you shower, then use a tablespoon of conditioner or Lemon Aid (see page 55) to cleanse your scalp and hair. Rinse thoroughly, and reapply conditioner as you normally would.

Try to wear a hat in the sun. It will protect your complexion, as well as your hair, from harmful ultraviolet rays.

A: I love the way my hair looks at the beach—the combination of sea salt and ocean breeze is a tonic for my curls. The sea salt is good for your hair, so don't rush to rinse it off. The salt helps separate the curls and gives them definition, and the breeze helps your hair dry faster, so the frizz factor is reduced. Bring a leave-in conditioner with sunblock in a spray bottle and spray your hair after you get out of the ocean. At the end of the day, follow the conditioning routine described on page 94 to keep your hair hydrated.

Watery Beginnings

I often have the fantasy that curly girls are mermaids who have had to adapt to life on dry land. We come from the sea. The ocean is in our blood. It sings through our heart and lungs, our skin and hair. Our curls require the nourishment only a watery environment can provide. Both ocean waves and curly hair are forces of nature that can't be tamed. We can only accept and admire their power and beauty.

I often borrow from the vocabulary of the ocean when I talk about curls. Like the waves in our hair, ocean waves form consecutive *C*'s. The highest point of a wave is the crest or peak; the lowest part is called the trough. Tossed by the wind and the elements, the ocean waves ebb and recede like our curls expanding and receding according to the dictates of the weather and our states of mind. We can never transform their essential properties.

Being near the ocean feels like coming home to curly girls. Our hair and ourselves thrive at the seashore. The combination of salt, wind, and water is a gift from the sea, a beckoning spray that feeds our curls and revives memories of our long-forgotten origins.

Q: How do I prevent hat hair?

A: Some curly girls think that wearing hats will make hair both flat and frizzy. But in fact, hats can reduce frizz; they act as a hairnet and keep hair in place as it dries. Before you put on your hat, use one of the pin tricks (see page 36) to keep the roots lifted.

When you take your hat off, loosen the curls by bending over, shaking your head a little, then fluffing them from underneath. To give the top layer of hair a quick lift, pick out a few of the flattened curls and spritz lightly with lavender spray or water. Twist each section around your index finger, then slide the curl off and either pin or hold it in place with your fingers for a couple of minutes. (If water isn't available, just lick your finger to create the proverbial spit curl.)

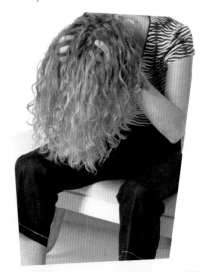

Q: I'm going through menopause. Can the hot flashes and night sweats negatively affect my hair?

A: While hot flashes may feel strange or uncomfortable, curly hair can actually benefit from the extra moisture that you're suddenly producing. Sweat, as I've said earlier, is salt water, a part of the body's ecosystem and a natural cleansing agent. If the hot flashes are especially frequent or severe, you may want to wear your hair up, especially in situations when you feel you need to keep your cool. Be sure to carry a travel-size bottle of Lavender Mist (see page 53) in your bag and car for a quick refreshing spritz to your hair, face, neck, or wherever you need it.

Q: I'm having a bad hair day. Help!

A: *There's no such thing as a bad hair day.* Okay, I'll admit that some days are more challenging than others. You're rushing off first thing in the morning and forget to put in enough conditioner or gel. A strong gust of wind disturbs the topography of your perfectly well-defined curls. You go shopping, try on lots of sweaters, and leave the dressing room with your hair flying out in all directions. What do you do, short of plopping on a hat or pulling the curls back in a ponytail?

Spritz your hair with water or lavender spray, wrap a few curls around your finger for a couple of minutes, and clip them at the roots. You've restored your curls and re-created your hairdo.

Here's another "quick save" trick: Bend your head so that your hair falls forward. Place your fingers about an inch from the roots and give the bottom layer of hair a quick shuffle so that it reconnects with the canopy. Decide you can feel okay today about a slightly wilder style. Notice how much positive feedback you get from friends—and strangers. You're a curly girl, so even if your hair isn't behaving the way you'd want it to, love your curls and wear them proudly.

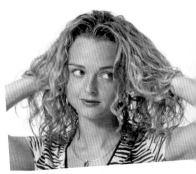

Fluffing from beneath

When I was little, my mother cut my hair very short—just two inches all over—so we wouldn't get into so many fights when she brushed it. I lived with that Bozo hair until second or third grade. It was the 1980s, and everyone had feathered hair. **I wanted to look like Daisy in *The Dukes of Hazzard.*** So I asked a hairdresser to feather mine. She layered both sides, which just made the curls tighter and frizzier and I looked like I was wearing earmuffs. It was mortifying. (Now I know enough about curly hair to never let a hairdresser layer my hair.)

Today I let my curls grow out, but if my hair gets wet and dries without conditioner, it will still frizz up and look like a dandelion gone to seed. Not a good look.

—**HEATHER CONWAY-VISSER, GRAPHIC DESIGNER**

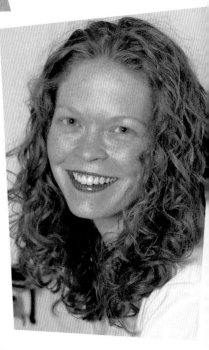

Q: My hair sometimes looks stringy, not curly. Is this from too much product or what?

A: You're probably applying too much conditioner to the ends, which absorb products less readily because they're older. Also, combing your hair unnecessarily can cause a stringy, noodle-like appearance.

Try scrunching with a spritz of Lavender Mist (see page 53) instead, and you'll probably see a change. If your ends still appear to be weighed down, they may need a trimming.

Q: How can I reduce the number of products I use and simplify my hair routine?

A: Not only do all the bottles and jars take up shelf space, but they can lead to a vicious cycle of product abuse. You become more and more dependent on an ever-expanding assortment of treatments and products, instead of caring for your curls with a simple, natural routine. Resist the urge to buy new products that promise hair greatness.

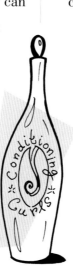

Now that you've learned how to care for your curls, you can liberate yourself by throwing out most of the bottles and jars gathering dust in the bathroom. Reduce your collection to three simple basics: a conditioner (instead of shampoo), an herbal cleanser, and a styling gel. Our curls need very little more than TLC and moisture to flourish and look beautiful.

Q: I'm very rushed in the morning. Do I need to wet my hair every day?

A: Your hair will tell you whether or not it needs a daily dose of water to look its best. Some curly girls report that wetting their hair once every two or three days works fine for them. (This is almost never true for Corkscrew curly girls.) You be the judge. Remember, hair care is voluntary, but if you feel you don't have time even for a quick spritz in the morning, you may want to reevaluate your schedule—or your self-image.

Q: I travel a lot. How do I protect my hair from the changes in climate and water?

A: Your hair is a natural weather barometer, so trust what it tells you. Adjust your hair care routine, depending on where you are and how your curls are responding. You may need less conditioner in Los Angeles, because the weather is generally dry; more in England, where the frequent drizzle and fog can bring out the frizzies in even the best-behaved curls. Don't leave home without your conditioner and herbal spray, both of which will see you through almost any climatic situation. (In a pinch your conditioner can also substitute as hand cream or body lotion and vice versa.) Be sure to pack some herbal spray in your carry-on bag to hydrate your skin *and* quench thirsty curls on long flights. The friendly skies are never forgiving to your locks.

Q: What is clarifying shampoo or rinse, and does it restore shine?

A: You've obviously figured out by now that I don't put much faith in shampoos. I have even less confidence in specialty products such as après-pool or clarifying shampoos and conditioners. These products are merely another way to sell you more of what you've already bought and are often even harsher on the hair than regular shampoo. They strip your hair of any hydration, whether your own or that from the conditioner you use. Don't waste your money on one more cleverly packaged product that will inevitably wind up in the garbage.

A: Any of the above, alone or in combination, can have a profound effect on your curls. As a nonessential organ, your hair is at the bottom of the physiologic hierarchy, so it's likely to be neglected by the body when the immune system is fighting disease or depression. Even the mildest medications may have side effects, and your hair is not immune to these reactions. One client swears that when she takes decongestants for a day or two, her normally bouncy curls get dry and flat.

An emotional crisis can often result in à breakout of hives, pimples, or cold sores. It shouldn't be a surprise, then, if your scalp and hair also reflect your emotional state. If you lose your job or break up with your boyfriend, you're likely to eat badly, stay up too late, and lie in bed instead of exercising.

Your hair will bounce back as soon as you do. In the meantime, keep it tied back lightly, don't skimp on conditioner, drink plenty of water, and, above all, don't make any drastic changes in your hairstyle. Wait until you're recovered to experiment with a new cut or a different color. If you don't feel well, your hair won't look good, no matter what you do to it.

A: No, not if your intention is to straighten it. But if the weather is frigid, and you're in a rush to leave the house, you can use a blow-dryer with a diffuser, or a travel hair dryer, on the "low" setting. Dry slowly to protect your hair from singeing or getting overheated.

A: Curly hair reacts strongly to every change in atmospheric conditions, whether it's high or low humidity, rain, sun, sleet . . . As humidity rises, very dry curls (especially the corkscrew variety) begin to move out in an east-west direction. On rainy or high-humidity days, be sure to wet your hair thoroughly, rather than giving it a quick spritz, and experiment with using extra conditioner. The additional residue will help pull your hair down and keep it moving south instead of east-west. And don't linger too long in a steamy bathroom after showering.

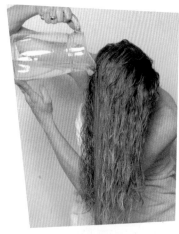

A cool rinse seals cuticles.

Another frizz-buster I recently discovered is giving curls one last cool rinse to seal the cuticles before styling. Fill a bowl with cool water or seltzer and dunk your head in after you get out of the shower. Towel-dry as much of the moisture as possible, then put about half a teaspoon of gel on the canopy to keep it smooth. Don't touch your hair once you've applied the gel, no matter how tempted you are to pat the strands into place. This is a general rule for curly girls that becomes particularly important on frizz-prone days.

If you have a special date or meeting, you can protect your locks and encourage your curls to swell to their natural state by *loosely* covering your head with a light scarf for about ten minutes after you've finished styling your hair.

One more thought on the subject of frizz: It is not necessarily a bad

After chemically relaxing my hair for so many years, going curly was a life-transforming experience. I've learned to love my curls rather than be afraid of them. I've saved myself so much time and heartache in the morning, and I no longer hate my hair. **I've become such a huge advocate of curly hair that any time I see a curly girl, I make a beeline to her and say, "I have to tell you what I know!"** Then I'll tell her about how I wash and dry it, about the bobby pin trick—they always appreciate this.

For me, there's no turning back from being a curly girl. Sometimes I'll see girls with cute pixie cuts and wish I could carry off that hairstyle. But then I'll think to myself, that's okay, they'll never be able to wear their hair long and curly, like mine.

All my life I've been the tall girl with dark curly hair and I've *finally*, happily come to terms with it. **I love my crazy, tight, banana curls— straight hair just isn't me.**

I know that sometimes during pregnancy one's hair can change dramatically. I dread the possibility that someday my hair might lose its curl.

—**TRACY KESSLER**, PRODUCER OF LIVE ENTERTAINMENT EVENTS

thing. I personally prefer a gentle halo of frizz around my head to stick-thin, petrified curls so coated with product that they remain stationary when you move your head. As an advanced curly girl (and I have clients who feel similarly), I think that if hair is healthy and the curls are basically well defined, frizzy can be sexy. I've received so many compliments on days when I haven't fought the frizz that I now accept it as one of the ways in which my curls sometimes choose to express themselves.

Q: Why does the front of my hair never seem to grow as long as the back?

A: Nothing frames a face better than a few shorter, curly locks of hair. The hair around your face is a protective barrier for the rest of your hair. It is constantly exposed to wind, rain, heat, and other environmental factors, and therefore it has a shorter life span. So don't be surprised if you can't grow out your bangs past your chin.

However, you can mend and protect the tendrils around your face by treating them gently and nurturing them with extra doses of conditioner. Pay attention to the damage you may be inflicting unwittingly. Are you constantly pulling your hair, twirling your bangs, or running your fingers through the strands? Always handle hair with care, and *only when absolutely necessary.*

Q: Why are my bangs so hard to control, and how do I encourage the curls to emerge?

A: Many curly girls complain of problem bangs. Let me be perfectly frank: your bangs will never lie flat. Accept the fact that a Louise Brooks "fringe" on the forehead is not in your future. However, it is possible to have funky, cropped bangs, or two or three curls that form a kind of bang, to frame and soften your face. Be sure to have your bangs cut dry, and never cut them straight across. Between the sunlight, wind, rain, blasts of hot air from the oven, and cold air from the

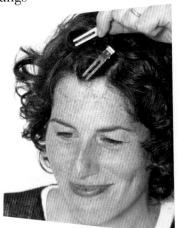

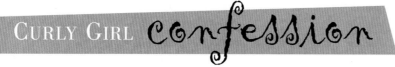

M y hair is on the frizzy side of curly. I wore it in pigtails when I was growing up, then blow-dryers came out and changed my life. I'd blow-dry my hair for forty-five minutes a day, five times a week. It was the seventies, and if I didn't do that, it would get bushy and stick out. I had lots of split ends. My sister would wrap my hair in orange juice cans. **I wore it long and straight, parted in the middle, trying for that Gloria Steinem look.** We had a swimming pool, but I'd never go swimming. It would ruin my hair.

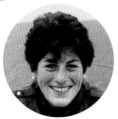

Then I went to England, to study history at Oxford, and I cut my hair very short—two inches all around. At Oxford, what you looked like said less about you than it does here. I really played with my hair there. I even dyed it pink.

Now, I love the fact that my hair is curly. Hairdressers still say, "It's too bushy, you need to go shorter or have it blown straight." But I ignore them. My daughter, who's four, has curly auburn hair. It's incredible. **I must have done something right: she loves her curls.**

—FRAN KELLNER, LAWYER

freezer, the hair around the forehead is the most delicate and weakest, so be kind to your bangs with regular conditioning. Finally, if your bangs simply aren't behaving one day, use the pin curl trick to keep them bouncy and well defined. Pull a curl out and place it where you want it. Put a clip at the root to hold it in place for a few minutes. Spray with water or a spray gel. Be patient. When it's dry, carefully remove the clip.

Q: How can I get rid of static?

A: Most curly girls don't have much of a static problem, once they throw away the hairbrush, use plenty of conditioner, and either eliminate or cut way back on shampoo.

If you do have severe static, however, I recommend using static-cling sheets: yes, the kind you throw in the clothes dryer. Pat gently across the top layer of your hair, and the static will disappear.

Q: Should I do anything special to my hair before I go to sleep at night?

A: If your hair is long, tie it back lightly to reduce tangling. You may sometimes also add extra conditioner or apply one of the moisturizing treatments I've suggested and leave on overnight. If so, be sure to use an old pillowcase or towel so as not to stain your regular cases with oil.

On other nights, use a sateen pillowcase or one with a high thread count to reduce friction and minimize split ends. The softer and more luxurious the cotton, the less damage it will do to your hair. And you may sleep better, too!

Q: What's the best way to tie back or put my curly hair in a ponytail without causing breakage?

A: Use a "scrunchie"—a ponytail holder that's covered with fabric—hair sticks or chopsticks, or a leather-covered clasp held in place with wooden sticks. Never use rubber bands or any other kind of elastic that could tug or tear your hair.

Tied in a Knot

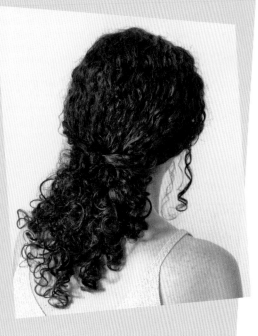

Tie your curls back *with* your curls. To get hair off your face or for end-of-the-day-hair-droop, try this pretty solution.

First pull your hair back. Take a one-inch section of hair from behind each ear. Cross the two strands over the rest of your hair and tie. Then pull a couple of curls out around the front, to frame your face.

Q: I know I have to give up the blow-dryer habit, but I'm afraid that if I go natural, my hair will look terrible. How long will it take before my curls start to look good?

A: If your hair is wavy, you'll see more curls within three weeks; if you're a Botticelli or Corkscrew, you'll notice a difference in less time, possibly within two weeks. Although your hair will love going natural, *you* yourself may need some time to get used to your new look. Get over the notion that your hair will bend to your will.

Learn what it wants and needs to look good—maybe more gel on a humid day or more conditioner in the winter. Your curls will look great even if they don't conform to your exact vision. Trust me, that vision will change as you acknowledge that you're a curly girl. After all, if you don't accept who you are, how do you expect others to?

Chapter Eleven

LOOKS FOR SPECIAL OCCASIONS

Easy Updos

I usually wear my hair down, because after so many years of hating my hair and feeling unattractive, I love to flaunt my curls. It's another way of telling the world that I'm proud to be a curly girl. I also enjoy the sensation of ringlets bouncing against my neck and around my face. But some days I wake up in the mood for something different, whether it's because the weather is hot and sticky or because I'm going out to dinner and want my hair to project that "special occasion" aura.

Your ringlets also have the unique ability to be delicately sculpted and piled high on your head. A simple updo will stay better—and endure for a longer period of time—on curly hair than on straight.

The first rule in any updo is to not over do. If a few extra ringlets fall out, leave them—an updo should show off your curls. Though ribbons, barrettes, and clips may dress up your hair beautifully, your natural curls will make any updo look romantic and classy.

Here are a few simple updos that are sexy, playful, funky, and, best of all, easy to create. Use caution when handpicking and parting the hair. You don't want to create snarls or knots.

Building a Foundation

Any secure building needs a foundation. When creating an updo, the same rule holds true. This technique gives you a solid base for the following two hairstyles, and it works for most hair lengths.

To build your base:

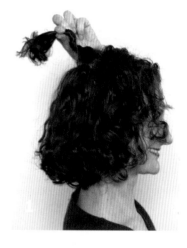

1. Part hair loosely in the center of the crown. Take a one-inch section of hair from the back of the crown (where your part ends). Lift it up and away from your crown, twisting firmly toward the forehead.

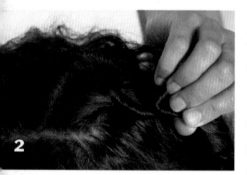

2. Roll the piece of hair around itself and into a tight, round coil.

3. Secure the first bobby pin diagonally, across the twist; then secure the second bobby pin so that it forms an *X* across the first pin. The coil will stand out quite a bit from the scalp, which will give your updo some nice height at the crown. Now you're ready to build up from your base.

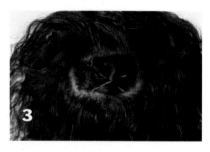

The "It" Curl

This romantic look for Botticelli curls works best with shoulder-length hair. Wait until your hair is dry and you've built a foundation (see facing page).

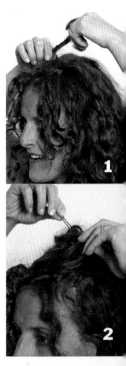

1. Beginning on one side of the part, pick up a small section of hair that falls in front of your ear, twist it firmly, starting at the root, all the way down to the end.

2. Bring the twist up so that it lies against or near your foundation. Secure it in place with a bobby pin. Repeat as above on the other side of your head.

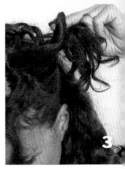

3. Bring the twist up so that it meets the first section. Secure this piece with one or two bobby pins.

You may stop at this point for a simple version or continue with as many pieces as you'd like, building in "twos" (i.e., one section of hair from each side of your part). Gently tease out a couple of curly tendrils just at the hairline on both sides of your forehead, to create a soft, sexy frame for your face.

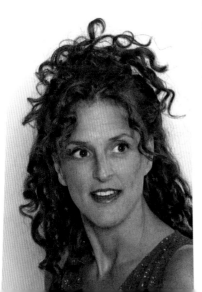

Curls' Night Out

For chin-length Botticelli or Wavy girls. With the variations below, this style can easily go from funky and tousled for day to a sexy after-hours look. First build your base (see page 110).

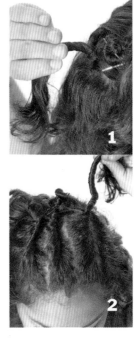

1. Beginning in the front at the hairline, twist a one-inch piece of hair back and away from your face. Continue making a loose, flat twist until it is possible to pin it to the foundation.

2. Repeat on the opposite side. Continue, working with equal amounts of hair from both sides of your head, until you've completely pinned up the top layer of hair.

3. Now take one-inch pieces from the nape of your neck, this time twisting up toward the top of your head.

4. Pin each piece at the crown but leave the ends loose. (Use two pins to keep your updo extra secure.) Pull a few ringlets out from the sides, near your ears, to frame your face.

You may want to clip a pretty barrette at the top to complete the look. Or, be a princess for the evening and don a tiara atop your crowning glory of curls.

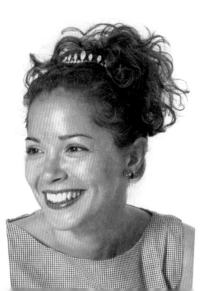

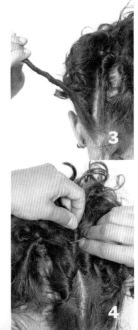

Corset Curls

[or Viking Maiden Meets Native American Princess]

This grown-up version of a ponytail works best on long-haired Botticelli or Wavy girls. Use a thin thread of black leather, about eighteen to twenty inches long and one-quarter to one-half inch wide, for an edgy, sexy, downtown look.

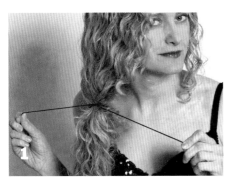

1. Gather hair gently to one side and pull over your shoulder. Tie a piece of leather around once and knot, to create a ponytail. You can make a tie at the nape or lower, at the collarbone.

2. Crisscross the leather down and around the hair to make a series of *X*'s. At about two inches from the ends of the curls, tie the leather and let the ends fall free.

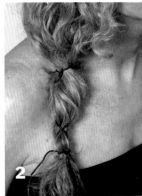

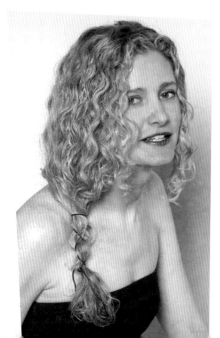

Knot for Everyone

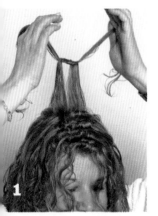

This top-knot style looks great on all curly girls—Corkscrew, Botticelli, and Wavy. The knots create an eye-catching texture and keep your hair out of your face.

1. While hair is fairly damp (or moistened with lavender spray), part in the middle. Take a one-inch strand of hair from each side of the part. Lift straight up and, as if tying a shoelace, knot once but don't tie completely.

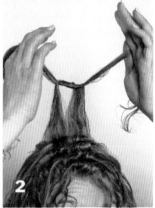

2. Next, pass each strand through once more to create a kind of rolled knot at the crown. Do this by bringing the left strand through (from back to front) and the right strand through (from front to back).

3. Now complete the knot by pulling the ends tight. I find that three or four top knots in a row look best, but you can tie fewer or more.

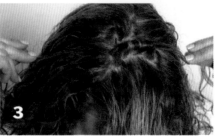

Goddess Curl

For long-haired girls with Corkscrew curls, this goddess updo is a great look when you're in the mood for something different. It can be dressed up for evening by following the suggestions on the next page.

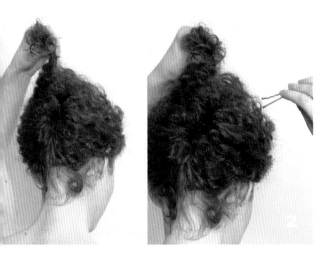

1. Gather your hair at the nape of the neck and twist it gently, rolling the twist inward up the back of your head in the direction of the crown. This creates a crease or seam in the back. When you've twisted the strands as far as they will reach, hold your hair in place with one hand.

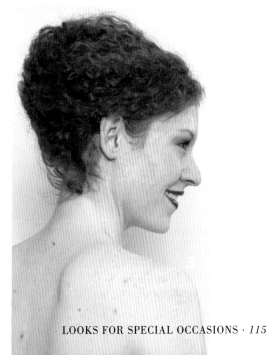

2. With your free hand, secure the twist to your crown by inserting two bobby pins in an *X*-shape at the top of the crease of the twist.

3. You may need to use several more bobby pins to weave the crease of the twist into the hair at your crown. Separate out a few of the curls to soften the look.

If you have short hair, follow the instructions above, but make the twist very tight, and use as many bobby pins as you need to secure the shorter strands of hair.

For a romantic twist on the "Goddess Curl," take a strand of colored ribbon or leather, lay it flat just behind the hairline so it looks like a head- band, and twist it around your head.

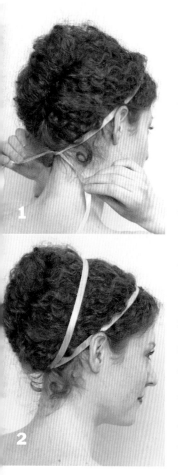

1. Make a knot at the back of your neck, crisscross twice around the chignon, and bring the ends up to cross at the top of your head.

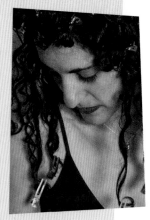

2. Knot or pin the ribbon in place with tiny sequined clips, leaving the ribbon to hang free. Or dress it up by inserting a fresh or dried flower at the side where the twist meets your crown or in the crease of the chignon.

Weight a Minute

How many times has this hap- pened to you? You're about to go out for the evening, but it's humid and your curls have contracted to a third their normal length, and your best friend, who should know better, asks you whether you just got a haircut, because "Your hair looks so much shorter."

If you notice as your hair is drying that your curls are shrinking, attach a hair clip to the bottom of your curls at the back of your head and the sides for five or ten minutes.

You can also attach the clipped hair to your shirt or sweater. (It may sound silly, but it works.) The weight of the clip will stretch out the strand and naturally reduce the spring factor.

Nip 'n' Tuck

Sometimes it's fun to go short. If you're not willing to commit to a cut, fake it with a fetching faux bob, circa 1920s. This 'do works best on shoulder-length or longer curls.

1. Pull all of your hair back as if putting it in a ponytail. Wrap an elastic band around the gathered hair about 1½ to 2 inches from the ends.

2. Next, roll the tail under to whatever "length" you prefer. It will look best just around chin level.

3. Secure the hair with at least four bobby pins, using the crossover technique, and fasten under the hair, at the nape of your neck.

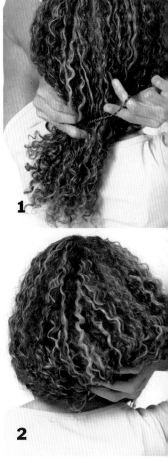

1

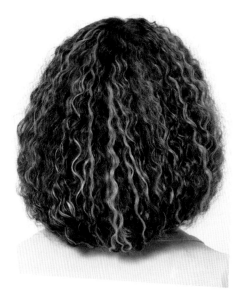

2

The Braided Bunch

For younger curly girls of any age or curl type, this style gives you lots of color and texture and it lasts for days. All you need is several spools of strong thread, either in bright, funky colors or in a shade that's close to your own hair color.

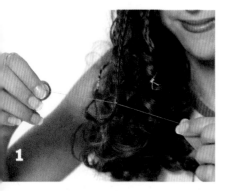

1. Cut a piece of thread about a foot long, halve it, and tie the two halves together in a knot. Choose a section of hair at random from the top of your head and braid it. Twist the thread around the bottom of the braid and tie it in a double knot.

2. For a fun variation: After braiding, tie the thread in a knot at the top of the braid, as close as possible to your scalp. Wind the thread around the length of the braid, finishing it off at the bottom with several wraps around the ends. Finally, tie the thread in a knot to secure. You can do several of both kinds for a funky, spring look.

Chapter Twelve

A 12-STEP RECOVERY PROGRAM FOR CURLY GIRLS

One Shampoo at a Time

It's not enough to admit that you're not straight; the compulsion to abuse products and your precious locks is deep seated and hard to shake. To help curly girls in recovery, we've invented a 12-step Personal Hair Growth and Recovery Program. Since sharing is a necessary part of the program, curly girls are advised to shift their obsession from product abuse to telling others about their curly conversion. When you feel the urge to shampoo or even brush your hair, stop first and call a friend.

The following steps are to be used only as life styling tools. Interpret them in the way that is most helpful to you personally and then follow them religiously. They have worked for millions of others who knew they were not straight. They can work for you. In the process of recovering your curls, you may recover other parts of yourself long since forgotten.

I ADMIT THAT I AM POWERLESS OVER MY TRUE NATURE—AND THAT MY CURLY HAIR WILL CONTINUE TO BE UNMANAGEABLE IF I DENY AND ABUSE IT AS I HAVE IN THE PAST.*

* You can fight the truth for only so long. Make peace now, stop deluding yourself, and see your hair for what it truly is.

I WILL STOP TORTURING MYSELF WITH BLOW-DRYERS, BRUSHES, STRAIGHTENERS, ROLLERS, IRONS, AND OTHER DIABOLICAL WAYS TO STRAIGHTEN MY HAIR, AND I WILL REGAIN MY SANITY AS A CURLY-HAIRED PERSON. I WILL SEARCH MY BATHROOM FOR SUCH ITEMS AND DONATE THEM TO CHARITY OR SELL THEM ON EBAY.

I WILL ADMIT MY ADDICTION TO GOING STRAIGHT AND ATTEMPT TO DISCOVER WHY I HAVE WASTED MY TIME IN THIS PURSUIT. I WILL ACCEPT THE NATURE OF MY HAIR AND CELEBRATE IT RATHER THAN FIGHT IT.

I WILL MAKE A DECISION TO TURN MY CURLS OVER TO A HIGHER POWER—THE POWER THAT CREATED ME AND MY HAIR—AND I WILL FIND A SPONSOR TO MENTOR ME AS A RECOVERING CURLY GIRL.

Step Five

I WILL GIVE IN TO THE FORCES OF NATURE, EMBRACING HUMIDITY, RAIN, AND WIND, FACING THE ELEMENTS CONFIDENTLY BECAUSE I AM NO LONGER ATTEMPTING TO GO AGAINST NATURE AND CONTROL MY CURLS.

Step Six

I WILL MAKE A LIST OF RELATIVES AND FRIENDS WHO ENCOURAGED MY CURL DENIAL WITH COMPLIMENTS ABOUT MY STRAIGHT HAIR. I WILL FORGIVE THEM AS WELL AS HAIRDRESSERS WHO ABETTED MY HABIT.

Step Seven

I WILL ACCEPT THAT THE SCALP AND THE HAIR ARE TWO DIFFERENT ORGANS WITH TOTALLY DIFFERENT NEEDS, AND I WILL TREAT EACH ACCORDINGLY.

Step Eight

I WILL GIVE UP FOREVER SHAMPOO DEPENDENCY AND LEARN HOW TO KEEP MY HAIR CLEAN WITHOUT TURNING TO PRODUCTS THAT HARM ME.

Step Nine

I ADMIT THAT IT IS MY RESPONSIBILITY TO TAKE CARE OF MY HAIR IN THE BEST WAY POSSIBLE. I WILL LEARN HOW TO DRY IT WITHOUT HARMING IT, AND I WILL LET MY CURLS GROW TO THEIR FULL POTENTIAL.

Step Ten

WHENEVER I AM TEMPTED TO GO STRAIGHT, I WILL CALL A MENTOR OR FRIEND WHO HAS EMBRACED HER CURLY DESTINY AND SEEK HER ENCOURAGEMENT IN LIVING AN HONEST CURLY LIFE.

Step Eleven

I WILL CARRY THE MESSAGE OF CURLY HAIR TO OTHER WOMEN STILL LIVING IN CURL DENIAL.

Step Twelve

I WILL PRACTICE THE PRINCIPLES THAT I HAVE LEARNED EVERY DAY OF MY LIFE.

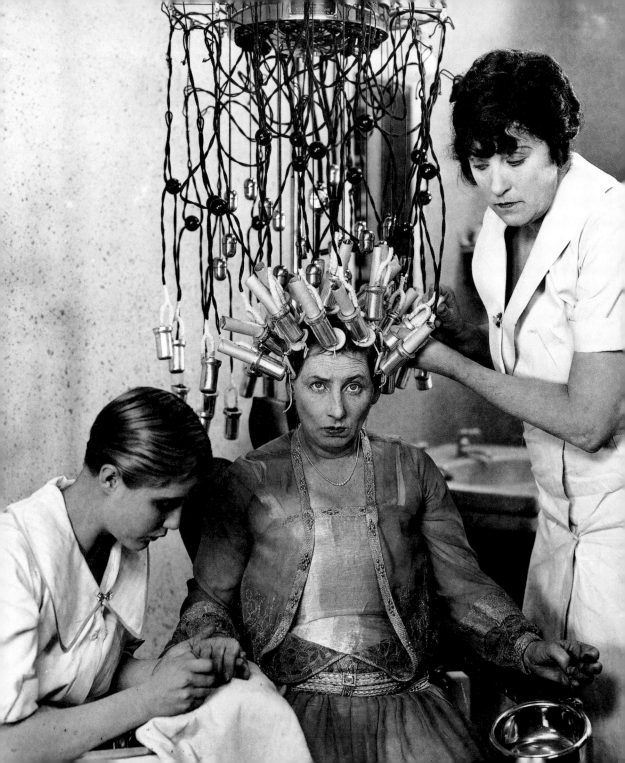

TIME LINE
A Cavalcade of Curls

IN THE BEGINNING

Curls are God-given and divine. There were no bad hair days in Paradise.

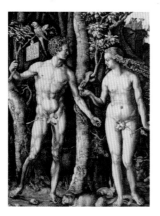

CURLS ON HIGH

Artists through history have depicted angels with curly hair. They are probably right. Curls are celestial.

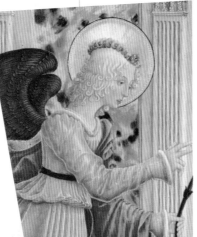

GODLY CURLS

All the Greek and Roman gods had curls—from the sculpted marble locks of the Apollo Belvedere (in the Vatican) to the fusilli curls of **Botticelli's *Venus*** in the fifteenth century. Diana, goddess of the hunt and the moon, was especially

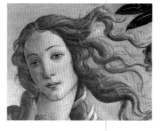

honored for her curly head. Women washed their hair once a year—on Diana's birthday, August 13.

2000 B.C.: ANCIENT EGYPT

Archaeologists have found evidence in Egypt of hairpins, combs, and curlers being used as far back as 2000 B.C. The curlers could create crimps (for fullness) or curls (for beauty). Curling irons and contraceptives were introduced around the same time, which makes sense. Curling tongs in the British Museum that date from the fifteenth century B.C. have attached blades—for trimming split ends.

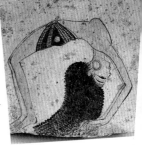

The upper classes wore wigs decorated with elaborate braids and curls, and arranged like tiles or puffed out into beehives. Their tightly plaited wigs resembled some popular contemporary African

American hairstyles, such as extensions and dreadlocks. The ancient Egyptians worried about frizz. But instead of Dippity-Do, hair was coated with beeswax and twisted around heated metal rods.

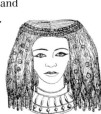

1500 B.C.: ANCIENT GREECE

The natural look was fashionable in Greece from 1500 to 650 B.C. Women wore their hair long, letting their curly locks cascade down to their shoulders in corkscrews or spirals. They used mud and pomades to "set" the curls, and ribbons and bands to hold them in place. The looks were amazingly contemporary.

70 B.C.: ANCIENT ROME

The Romans didn't begin to curl their hair or use wigs until about the third century B.C., when they started to copy the Greeks with great enthusiasm. Intellectuals found the trend ridiculous. "I will tear from your head those curly perfumed false locks you have so carefully arranged," says a character in one Plautus play.

But elaborate curls caught on. Around 70 B.C. Roman matrons were getting their hair curled with a device called a calamistrum—a hollow stick made of bronze. Ivory, gold, silver, and bone hairpins held the curls in place.

In the early part of the millennium, Roman women started wearing even more elaborate hairdos, arranging their phony curls around a crescent-shaped wire called an orbis. It was probably an attempt "to get some height," the same impulse that gave rise to the beehive—1,950 years later.

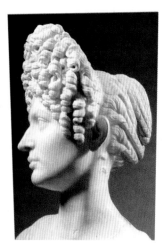

SECOND CENTURY A.D.: ROMAN EMPIRE

Hairstyles got more elaborate and thick, with false curls, expensive wigs, and hair dye (black or blond). These enhancements infuriated the early church fathers. St. Clement of Alexandria inveighed against all the "frizeling and curling of

Haire" and ruled that if you were wearing a wig when blessed, only the wig got the blessing. He was on to something— the barbarians were at the gates.

A.D. 500–1200: DARK AGES

They don't call these the Dark Ages for nothing. Few images remain. Many women kept their hair covered to show modesty.

In Byzantium, the head could be decorated with jewels. **Empress Theodora** is shown in mosaics with an elaborate headdress with beads shaped like long spiral curls. But you can't see her hair.

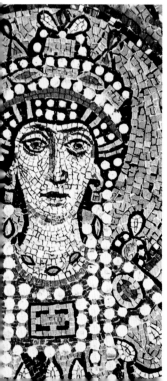

FOURTEENTH AND FIFTEENTH CENTURIES

Hair came out of the closet. A high forehead was a mark of beauty, so wealthy women plucked their foreheads and wore their hair in elaborate coiled braids, which disguised any natural curls. Sometimes hair was rolled, but curls were rare.

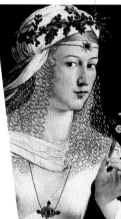

SIXTEENTH CENTURY

Queen Elizabeth I, who was bald, loved wigs of tight red curls. Mary Queen of Scots wore her tresses straight and smooth. She lost her head.

In the latter part of the century, wealthy women started waving and curling their hair. Even when they wore tight caps, they frizzed whatever hair was left showing. Curly wigs made a comeback.

SEVENTEENTH CENTURY

The Baroque era, excessive in all artistic expression, produced grandiloquent hairstyles. Wigs for women became more elaborate, although kings like Louis XIV could wear their naturally curly hair long and free.

In the first half of the century, women frizzed their hair for a fringe across the forehead, then used heated *bilboquets* or *roulettes* to curl their hair, letting the curls fall loose below a chignon or bun.

By the last half of the century, curls were so hot that a language of curls was developed, which

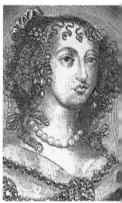

included the high curle, open curle, drake tail curle, and snake curle. Hair was frizzed or crisped. Women wore towers of false curls, called a *tour. Confidentes* were small curls near the ears, while *creve-coeurs,* or heartbreakers, were curls at the nape of the neck.

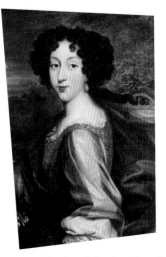

The **hurluberlu** (above) became the most popular hairstyle, both in England and in France. Madame de Sévigné thought she was too old for it but recommended it to her daughter. The hair was parted in the middle, then curled with short, fat ringlets all over the crown and sides. Some hair was left long so graceful locks could fall coyly down each side to the shoulders.

The *fontange,* in which the hair was piled extraordinarily high on the head, was invented by the **duchesse de Fontange,** who was sleeping with Louis XIV. Out hunting with Louis one day, the duchess lost her hat and tied up her curls with a lace-edged garter. Louis found this tousled look delightful and declared it the style of the moment. The duchess allegedly used a wire frame to hold it up and egg whites to keep the hair in place.

How did other women keep all these curls in place? One beauty book of the time advised making a paste with gum arabic and water, then using a curling iron. After mixing the ointment over a "gentle fire," you rubbed it on your hair for a style called "Curiously Curled." Indeed.

EIGHTEENTH CENTURY

Hair grew simpler for the first half of the century— Louis XIV had tired of his mistress and her hair. But hairdressers became so adept at constructing towers of hair that the fad came back with a vengeance in the last half of the century.

Hairdressers created towers of curls and filler— scraps of wool, flowers, pompoms, ribbons, feathers, pearls, even miniature ships. Legros de Rumigny, the Alexandre de Paris of his time, gave classes in Paris in the construction of such coiffures. He recommended beef fat as a pomade. Newspapers made fun of the styles and complained about the stench coming from hairdos that hadn't been changed for months. Mites and other vermin were reported escaping from the hairdos.

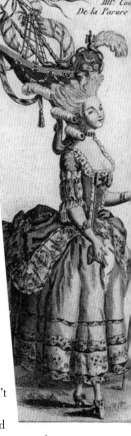

The height thing became ridiculous. Marie Antoinette, it was said, had

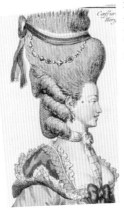

to remove her headdress before getting into her carriage. Other women just stuck their heads out the windows for the ride. As the hair grew higher, the curls took a backseat, although in England women had the ends of their hair frizzed in a style that was called **the hedgehog.**

Alas, at the end of the century, many of those hairdos came off, along with their owners' heads.

NINETEENTH CENTURY

For a time, inspired by the Revolution, Frenchwomen adopted short bobs, sometimes with their natural curls showing at the neck. The idea was to look as Republican as possible. Those evolved into Grecian styles—like the coif of **Madame Récamier,** a turn-of-the-century Parisian

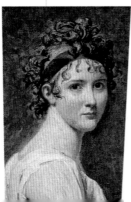

trendsetter whose hair was pulled up but softened with curls around the face. Women achieved this look with a fixative called "antique oil." If weather caused their stubborn tresses to lose their spring, they resorted to curly hairpieces.

In England, women let their ringlets fall naturally. Hair would be tied in a topknot or chignon, but spirals of curls would fall gracefully over the

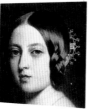

shoulders. Across the ocean, the elite adopted the same styles.

Eventually the topknot came down and women wore their hair smooth on top and cascading into long spirals, sausages of curls, or, like the young **Queen Victoria** (above), in coils of braids.

It became fashionable to have a lot of hair, so much so that, in 1848, Britain imported 8,766 pounds of French hair. Hair would be piled high on the head, with ringlets and

"frizettes" framing the face and trailing down the back.

Curls continued to be fashionable for the rest of the decade.

1852: THE MARCEL REVOLUTION

In 1852, a Frenchman named **Marcel Grateau** invented an instrument that changed the world. Rather than crimping the hair as past curling irons did, his instrument created soft, natural-looking waves. He called the effect moiré, or watered, undulations. But eventually his achievement

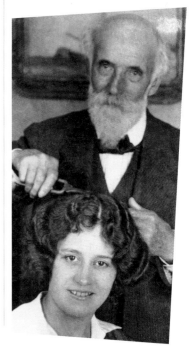

was named for him, and the marcel wave took hold for the next eighty or so years.

Grateau introduced a new simple style of soft, **Pre-Raphaelite** waves. Opera singer Nellie Melba and Caroline "La Belle" Otero, a famous actress of the period, would come to him for their marcels. Now the hair could be pinned up or pulled back, but soft, natural-looking waves could soften the effect.

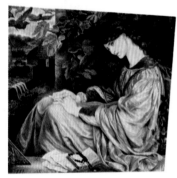

1900–1919: POMPADOURS AND GIBSON GIRLS

Hair was long but worn up in soft waves and curls, with fringes of bangs or a "rat," which was a roll of hair covered with an invisible hairnet that was placed high on the forehead and covered over with the

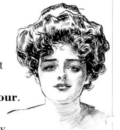

owner's natural hair. The result was a **pompadour**. The sides were softly waved with the marcel curling iron. **Gibson girls** frizzed curls on their foreheads.

1904: THE PERMANENT WAVE

A German named Karl Nessler devised an **electric permanent waving machine** in 1904, but it took twelve hours to get a permanent—and it was a huge contraption of a machine. The device didn't become popular until after World War I.

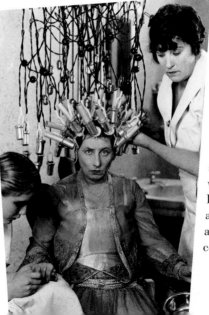

1920: THE BOB

When dancer **Irene Castle** bobbed her hair after the war, she set off the first major hair trend of the twentieth century. We think of the bob today as a short straight style. But in 1920, to bob your hair meant simply to cut it short. Whether it was curly or straight depended on your genetic inheritance. Women thronged to barbershops to be shorn. It was a boon for permanents. Many women felt they couldn't just have short straight hair—they'd look like men.

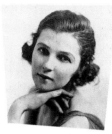

"The bob of today . . . is based on the wave," pronounced *Collier's* magazine in the 1920s. "Straight hair is something so infrequently seen that it must be classed as a personal idiosyncrasy." But short, neatly defined wavy hair—just like Irene's—was flattering and easy to wear. And accessible, if you could afford to get a permanent wave (which cost about $35 at the time).

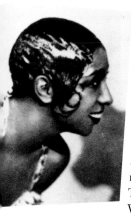

If you were a siren, say, like Wallis Simpson going after a king or like **Josephine Baker,** the toast of Paris, you affected ultra-sophisticated, almost sculpted marcel waves. The duchess of Windsor wore marcel waves for thirty years, finally adopting the bouffant in the 1960s. The look didn't require a permanent, just some well-placed wave clips inserted into the hair when it was still wet.

1930S

The curly or wavy bob look lasted for most of the 1930s. **Myrna Loy** in the *Thin Man* series, **Irene Dunne, Sylvia Sidney,** Rosalind Russell . . . all had curls, via permanent waves, nature, or pin curls.

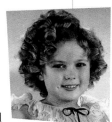

Meanwhile, a curly-headed **Shirley Temple** danced her way onto the stage and into the national consciousness, forever establishing curls as cute— but maybe not sophisticated anymore. Gradually, as the decade wore on, grown-up women let their hair grow a little longer. It was curly or not.

But then two movies changed everything. The first was *Gone With the Wind,* in which

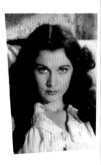

Vivien Leigh portrayed Scarlett with long and wavy raven tresses.

1940S

Then, in 1941, **Veronica Lake** (right), a sultry blonde with soft curls, appeared in a B movie called *I Wanted Wings.* Lake's signature S-shaped wave of hair covered one eye and fell

seductively to her shoulder. Suddenly everyone was attempting the look. Defense plants complained it was endangering Rosie the Riveter types, but the style persisted.

For most of the 1940s, hair was worn flat on top and parted on the side, falling gracefully into a few well-placed waves.

But **Rita Hayworth**'s long lanky look was mostly for younger women. Moms tended to wear short curly hair, regularly permed to perfection. The cold permanent wave was invented in 1947, and suddenly you could do it yourself. A lot of frizz and fumes resulted, but the hair was easy to maintain.

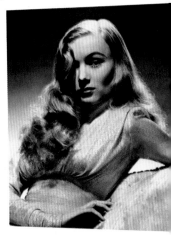

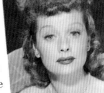

1950S

Curly hair dominated the first half of the decade, and **Lucille Ball**'s almost poodle-cut curls became a national institution. They went with Dior's "New Look": the long bouffant skirts and wasp waists required neat, sculpted hair with careful curls and waves.

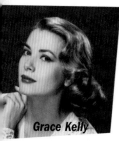
Grace Kelly

1960S

In the 1960s African Americans wore their hair in Afros as a political statement, and many women aspired to look like **Angela Davis** by letting their hair grow into 'fros.

But most white women's hairstyles were straight. Hippie men who couldn't be bothered let their hair frizz out like Albert Einstein's. Hippie girls tended to wear theirs natural and the longer the better.

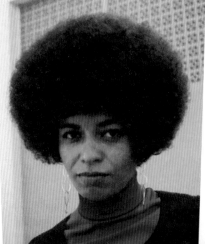

In 1961 Charles Schultz introduced curly-mopped **Frieda** into his *Peanuts* cartoon strip. While most girls in the '60s were trying to go straight, Frieda lived comic strip life by her inspired dictum: she could do anything because she had "naturally curly hair!"

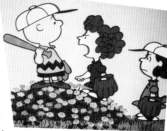

If you were chic and avant-garde, you copied Audrey Hepburn's existentialist pixie in *Funny Face* (1957) or adopted the gaminlike looks of Fellini's wife, **Giuletta Masina.**

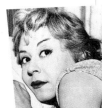

Less rebellious types ballooned up with beehives and bouffants. "Visible waves are absent," wrote *Chicago Tribune* fashion editor Eleanor Nangle in 1963, describing the latest trends in hairdressing, "and there isn't the trace of a curl."

Back-combing or teasing, which hadn't been seen since before the French Revolution, reappeared. Women with curly hair learned to iron it or blow-dry it out straight.

1970S

This was the decade that many curly girls still remember, in agony. They ironed their hair or rolled it in orange juice or beer cans to get it straight. The only possible variation was the **Farrah Fawcett** look—long and

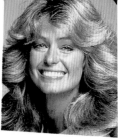

basically lanky, with feathery waves. These had to look phony; real curls wouldn't work.

1973: MOST HUMILIATING MOVIE MOMENT FOR CURLY GIRLS

A lot of curly girls still recall the movie moment that truly betrayed them and their hair. It was in *The Way We Were*, the 1973 movie starring **Barbra Streisand** and Robert Redford. In college, Barbra's character let her corkscrew curls go natural, and Redford never looked her way.

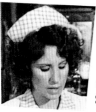

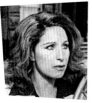

Cut to five years later: she's a knockout with ironed hair, and, yes, she got the guy. For some curly girls, Streisand didn't make up for this politically incorrect moment until 1983, when she proposed to a Botticelli-haired **Amy Irving** in *Yentl*. Barbra, who was

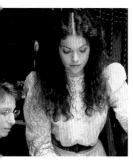

masquerading as a guy, hid her own curls in this one.

1980S

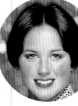

The **Dorothy Hamill** straight, short wedge was the most ubiquitous style of the early eighties, but renegades were starting to appear. Amy Irving in *Honeysuckle Rose* won Willie Nelson's heart with her Botticelli curls. And even Dyan Cannon, who'd straightened her hair for earlier movies, let her curls show in this one.

The 1980s was also the decade of "big hair"— you remember, the teased-and-sprayed, helmet-head, mall-mama thang.

1982

Cute curly carrot top **Orphan Annie** in the seventy-five-year-running comic strip appears in the

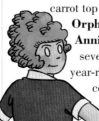

Broadway musical *Annie*. **Aileen Quinn** plays Annie in the film adaptation.

1990S

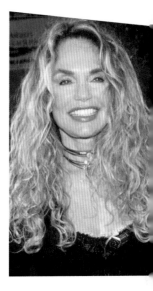

The pendulum swung the other way to hair that was flat and broomstick straight.

By the late 1990s stick-straight hair lost its cachet, and the new century is a curly millennium.

TV actresses with curls are making waves: **Dyan Cannon,** who had straight hair in 1969's *Bob & Carol & Ted & Alice*, is the definitive older curly girl of the millennium.

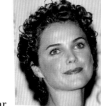

2000

When *Felicity* star **Keri Russell** lopped off all her curls, ratings for her show *Felicity* plummeted. The upshot: Russell's new contract with WB includes the proviso that she not cut

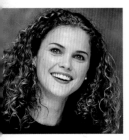

her hair for the duration of the show.

Suddenly everyone is clamoring for curls. The tide has turned, and everyone wants to catch the wave. Straight-haired women are resorting to pin curls and scrunch, rollers and permanent waves. It's finally our turn and it's about time.

2001 AND BEYOND

According to *InStyle* magazine, many celebrities, like **Sandra Bullock**, are faking the must-have look for spring—curly hair! "After their hair is curled," reports one stylist-to-the-stars, "they feel more flirty and feminine."

Curly girls protest the release of Disney's *The*

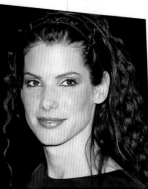

Princess Diaries, a modern fairytale flick that features an ugly duckling teenage girl who is transformed into a swan— via brush and blow-dryer. The founders of the Web site www.naturallycurly.com boycott the film.

"Hairstories" premieres at Jacob's Pillow in Becket, Massachusetts, by the **Urban Bush Women Dance Company**. Blending choreography, music, and videotaped interviews with black women, the show explores and celebrates the once pejorative

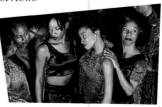

term *nappiness* and the culture that surrounds black women's hair.

The *Mademoiselle* September 2001 issue asked men to rate the hairstyles of fifty women. Among various lengths, straightnesses and textures, the curliest girl came in *first!* According to the judges, she looked the most "playful," "sexy," "chic," and "touchable."

Elle magazine features a cover story on the power of curls, along with information on curling your hair, using setting lotion, and scrunching. The headline:

UPWARD SPIRAL: THE SEASON'S MOST GLAMOROUS COIFS ARE ANYTHING BUT STRAIGHT. WHETHER TEASED, CURLED OR WAVED, MODERN HAIR IS FINALLY TAKING AN INTERESTING TURN.

We couldn't have said it better.

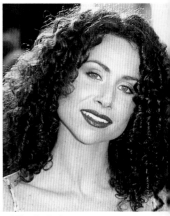

Minnie Driver

IT'S A CURLY WORLD

The curly hair look is *in!* All those celebrities with the natural ringlets are letting their hair go free. Curly girls are the ones to watch this season—from stars like Nicole Kidman, with her fabulous Botticelli ringlets, to Minnie Driver, whose cascading corkscrew curls turn heads and land roles, and Meg Ryan, whose tousled, sexy bed-head look has replaced Jennifer Anniston's as the look of the new decade. Below are just a few of the curly girls who have become fashion's new role models.

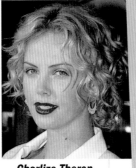

Meg Ryan

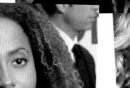

Nicole Kidman

nelope Cruz

Sarah Jessica Parker

Lisa Nicole Carson

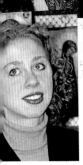

Chelsea Clinton

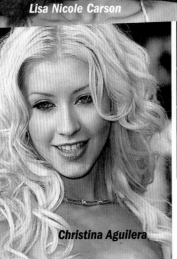

Christina Aguilera

Charlize Theron

Ananda Lewis

ASTROLOCURLS
A Horoscope

Aries
MARCH 21–APRIL 19

As spring stirs, the season of renewed life and the start of the sun's annual cycurl, fiery Aries symbolizes beginnings. You are full of fixed ideas, so your boundless curls may threaten you, to the point where you may butt heads with the herd. If you don't rise to the occasion, your hair will. Submit. After all, the part of the body ascribed to Aries is the head.

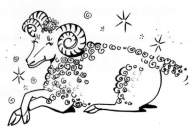

Taurus
APRIL 20–MAY 20

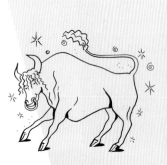

Taurus signals the rites of spring, and spring is in the hair. Taurus types who cultivate their gardens willingly may be inclined to get stuck in the mud and might dig in their heels and resist change as a result of many bad hair experiences. Don't be closed to new information. Seek a logicurl approach: you are known to be the goddess of the past. But don't be a has-been. Be the goddess of the now and try a new look.

Gemini
MAY 21–JUNE 21

Gemini brings in the mellow breezes of the summer—and, yes, with it, the humidity. As a twin, staring at your reflection, you have a need for individuality. But you have to accept that going straight and going curly is not always a heal-thy option. If your hair shows any sign of damage, you, as the embodiment of the quickening of human intelligence, must accept its truths. Once you get to know your hair's natural state, it will present itself differently every day. How can you be bored?

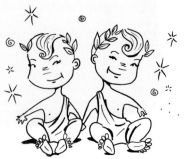

Cancer

JUNE 22–JULY 22

The sun has reached its highest point over the Northern Hemisphere. Open to new ideas, you must nevertheless set limits as a mother must for her adventuresome child. You do not readily accept others, so you may be in need of a worthy hairdresser to guide you right. Being moody with your hair won't solve a thing. Coexist; it's worthy of you. Curl up with *Curly Girl*, then pass it on to another Cancer curlfriend.

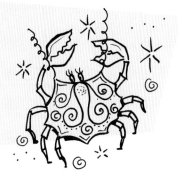

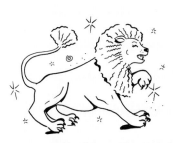

Leo

JULY 23–AUGUST 22

At the heat of the high summer, with its intense solar rays, curls are running rampant. It's time to explore your *S*-sence. When dealt with properly, your mane will inspire radiance and you will become a leader, encouraging other curly girls to emerge from their dens. If you deny your curls and slink off to try to smooth away the frizzies, by high noon, the untamed will of the frizz will persist.

Virgo

AUGUST 23–SEPTEMBER 22

At the beginning of the fall harvest, Virgo's humble awareness equips you early in life with an understanding of your hair's potential. But with your quest for perfection, you need to remember the old saying "It's not perfect, but it's perfect for you." Life's too short to be dissatisfied with one stray frizz. Look at the big picture, and stop fussing; otherwise you'll have big hair. Remember, while your hair is drying, do not micromanage.

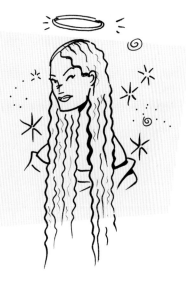

Libra

SEPTEMBER 23–OCTOBER 23

This is the fall equinox, when the sun enters the sign of Libra, a h'air sign that holds an invisible thread connecting us all. Libra rules relationship, one to one, and you are often one with your hair. If not, you may pay too much attention to the counsel of others and not be in touch with your inner curl. But you will eventually arrive at your hair's true state of harmony. With the right *Curly Girl* bible, you'll be one of us.

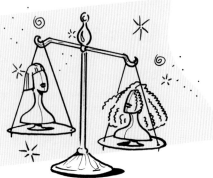

Scorpio

OCTOBER 24–NOVEMBER 21

As the nights grow longer, with a suggestion of winter, you consummate the bond with your hair with intense experimentation. Together, you must confront its *S*-sence in pursuit of the hairy truth. The unbound curl emerges and is understandably a challenge to pursue daily, weekly, monthly, yearly. Scorpio is attuned to the cycurl of death and rebirth, choosing to weather all weather conditions, since we have no choice in the realm of our hair. Scorpio tails will make your hair curl—if it's not already.

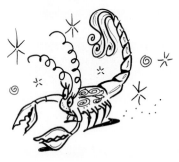

Sagittarius

NOVEMBER 22–DECEMBER 21

Born in the winter months, you Sagittarians need your hair to be as carefree and easy as you are, as long as you have a hair routine to follow. You sometimes come off sounding self-righteous, so lighten up, curlfriend. You're the perfect outreach curly girl, especially at holiday party time, since people are always asking you about your hair. It's all about your hair-itude, sweetie.

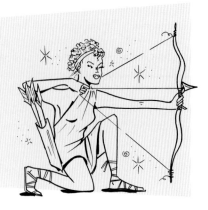

Capricorn

DECEMBER 22–JANUARY 19

Capricorn is born in the heart of winter, a product of the longest nights. Capricorns have their own particular vision of the world, so you may at first rebel against your curls. You typically need to be on top; you are determined to overcome all obstacles, and your hair may be one of them. Let down your guard, reach out to a curlfriend, and unite. Remember, your hair is on top, not you.

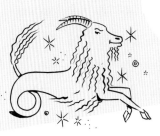

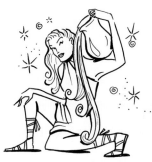

Aquarius

JANUARY 20–FEBRUARY 18

Aquarius is the ruler of the h'air wave. Winter has been too long, and as the water bearer, curls R U. You usually confront your hair frustrations, but if you're slightly insecure, you may demand that your hair change according to your perception of the situation. If you reject your curls, you reject your *S*-sense. Curl now, or forever hold your hair piece.

Pisces

FEBRUARY 19–MARCH 20

The days lengthen and thaws begin as Pisces moves beyond herself, always following the movement of the ocean currents and the current trends. You are easily swayed, which is both your strength and your weakness, and this trait also applies to your hair. Sometimes overwhelmed by what's current, you flounder in the face of your curly hairitage. If you can just ride the wave, you can be on top of anything.

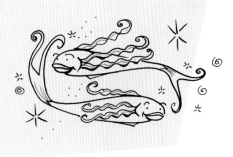

There was a little girl
Who had a little curl
Right in the middle of
    her forehead.
When she was good
She was very, very good,
But when she was bad,
    she was horrid.

—Henry Wadsworth Longfellow

Curly Diary

First curly haircut (date) _____

Day 1 _____

Day 2 _____

First week without shampooing _____

_____

_____

_____

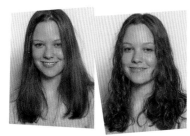

Gave away hairbrush and blow-dryer _____

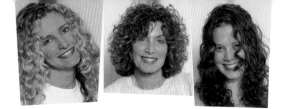

I found my inner curl. I am a:

Corkscrew ☐   Botticelli ☐   Wavy ☐

Comments about my new curls _____

_____

_____

_____

_____

_____

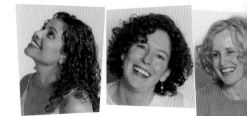

My curly hair makes me
feel like...

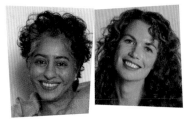

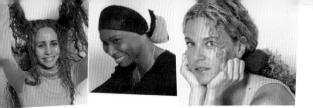

Bad hair day and how I coped

Number of days without shampooing

Saturday. Big date. Tried new homemade
conditioning recipe. How hair felt

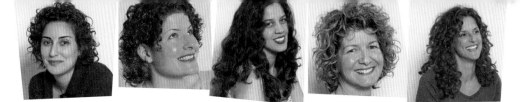

Boyfriend's (husband's) response to my new curls

Another curly girl asks for advice about caring for her curls

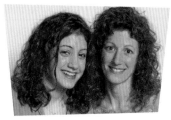

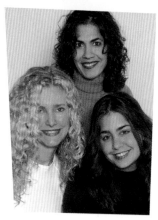

Curly girl support group

Let hair grow out for two months

Appointment with stylist. Her comments and suggestions

Four months since
last shampoo, but who's counting?

Photo Credits

Front cover: *(main image)* photographer/Güler Uğur, model/Heather Conway-Visser; *(top image)* Marc Dolphin/
Getty Images/Store; *(bottom)* Anthony Loew

Back cover: *(all)* Anthony Loew

Page iv: Photofest

Page vi: Photofest

Page viii: The Art Archive/Galleria Nazionale dell'Umbria Perugia/Dagli Orti

Page x: Tricia Meadows/Globe Photos

Page 11: Oliver Meckes/Photo Researchers, Inc.

Page 15: *(left)* John Durham/Science Photo Library/Photo Researchers, Inc.; *(right)* Biophoto Associates/
Photo Researchers, Inc.

Page 18: *(left)* John Spellman/Retna Ltd.; *(right)* Rose Hartman/Globe Photos

Page 20 *(left to right)*: Fitzroy Barrett/Globe Photos; Marion Curtis/DMI/Timepix; Steve Granitz/Retna Ltd.

Page 22 *(left to right)*: Tricia Meadows/Globe Photos; Marion Curtis/Timepix; AP/Wide World Photos

Page 24 *(left to right)*: Fitzroy Barrett/Globe Photos; Nina Prommer/Globe Photos; AP/Wide World Photos

Page 37: Photofest

Page 95: Kobal Collection/Gainsborough

Page 124: Photofest

Page 125: *(The Fall of Man)* Historical Picture Archive/Corbis Images; *(Archangel Gabriel)* The Art Archive/
Galleria Nazionale dell'Umbria Perugia/Dagli Orti; *(The Birth of Venus)* Erich Lessing/Art Resource;
(Egyptian Dancing Girl) Erich Lessing/Art Resource

Page 126: *(Vabia Matilda)* The Art Archive/Museo Capitolino Rome/Dagli Orti

Page 127: *(Empress Theodora)* The Granger Collection, New York; *(Bartolommeo Veneto)* The Granger Collection,
New York; *(Queen Elizabeth I)* Victoria and Albert Museum, London/Art Resource; *(Eleonore-Marie Louise)*
courtesy of the New York Public Library/Picture Collection

Page 128: *(Queen Marie-Louis)* The Art Archive/JFB; *(Marie Angelique Fontage)* courtesy of the NY Public Library/
Picture Collection; *(De la Parure des Dames)* courtesy of the New York Public Library/Picture Collection

Page 129: *(Hedgehog style)* The Art Archive/Musee Carnavalet Paris/Dagli Orti; *(Queen Victoria)* Giraudon/
Art Resource/NY; *(Juliette Recamier)* Erich Lessing/Art Resource; *(M. Marcel Grateau)* Hulton-Deutsch
Collection/Corbis Images

Page 130: *(Rossetti's La Pia)* Art Resource/NY; *(Karl Nessler)* Photofest; *(Irene Castle)* Photofest

Page 131: *(Josephine Baker)* CSU Archives/Everett Collection; *(Myrna Loy)* Photofest; *(Irene Dunne)* Photofest;
(Sylvia Sidney) Photofest; *(Shirley Temple)* Photofest; *(Vivien Leigh)* Photofest; *(Rita Hayworth)* Photofest;
(Veronica Lake) Photofest

Page 132: *(Lucille Ball)* The Kobal Collection; *(Grace Kelly)* The Kobal Collection; *(Peanuts cartoon)* Photofest;
(Giuletta Masina) Everett Collection; *(Angela Davis)* Corbis Images; *(Farrah Fawcett)* Everett Collection

Page 133: *(Barbra Streisand, both)* Photofest; *(Yentl)* Photofest; *(Dorothy Hamill)* Everett Collection; *(Annie)* Photofest;
(Annie, cartoon) Photofest; *(Dyan Cannon)* Mirek Towski/DMI/Timepix

Page 134: *(Keri Russell, left)* Armando Gallo/Retna Ltd.; *(Keri Russell, right)* Jerry Dabrowski/Zuma/Timepix;
(Urban Bush Women) Jennifer Lester/Urban Bush; *(Sandra Bullock)* Andrea Renault/Globe Photos;
(Minnie Driver) Corbis Outline

Page 135: *(Penelope Cruz)* Andrea Renault/Globe Photos; *(Chelsea Clinton)* Kevin Lamarque/Reuters/Archive Photos;
(Nicole Kidman) AP/Wide World Photos; *(Lisa Nicole Carson)* Mark J. Terrill/AP Photos; *(Christina Aguilera)*
Fitzroy Barrett/Globe Photos; *(Sarah Jessica Parker)* Tricia Meadows/Globe Photos; *(Charlize Theron)*
Fred Prouser/Reuters; *(Meg Ryan)* Nina Prommer/Globe Photos; *(Ananda Lewis)* Fitzroy Barrett/Globe Photos